Sedation and Sleep in Critical Care: An Update

Editor

JAN FOSTER

CRITICAL CARE NURSING CLINICS OF NORTH AMERICA

www.ccnursing.theclinics.com

Consulting Editor
JAN FOSTER

June 2016 • Volume 28 • Number 2

ELSEVIER

1600 John F. Kennedy Boulevard • Suite 1800 • Philadelphia, Pennsylvania, 19103-2899

http://www.theclinics.com

CRITICAL CARE NURSING CLINICS OF NORTH AMERICA Volume 28, Number 2
June 2016 ISSN 0899-5885, ISBN-13: 978-0-323-44652-5

Editor: Kerry Holland
Developmental Editor: Colleen Viola

Critical Care Nursing Clinics of North America (ISSN 0899-5885) is published quarterly by Elsevier Inc., 360 Park Avenue South, New York, NY 10010-1710. Months of issue are March, June, September, and December. Business and Editorial Offices: 1600 John F. Kennedy Blvd., Suite 1800, Philadelphia, PA 19103-2899. Periodicals postage paid at New York, NY and additional mailing offices. Subscription prices are $155.00 per year for US individuals, $370.00 per year for US institutions, $100.00 per year for US students and residents, $200.00 per year for Canadian individuals, $464.00 per year for Canadian institutions, $230.00 per year for international individuals, $464.00 per year for international institutions and $115.00 per year for Canadian and international students/residents. To receive student/resident rate, orders must be accompanied by name of affiliated institution, data of term, and the *signature* of program/residency coordinator on institution letterhead. Orders will be billed at individual rate until proof of status is received. Foreign air speed delivery is included in all *Clinics* subscription prices. All prices are subject to change without notice. **POSTMASTER:** Send address changes to *Critical Care Nursing Clinics of North America*, Elsevier Health Sciences Division, Subscription Customer Service, 3251 Riverport Lane, Maryland Heights, MO 63043. **Customer Service: 1-800-654-2452 (US and Canada); 314-447-8871 (outside US and Canada). Fax: 314-447-8029. E-mail:** JournalsCustomerService-usa@elsevier.com **(for print support) and** JournalsOnlineSupport-usa@elsevier.com **(for online support).**

Reprints. For copies of 100 or more of articles in this publication, please contact the Commercial Reprints Department, Elsevier Inc., 360 Park Avenue South, New York, New York, 10010-1710; Tel.: 212-633-3874, Fax: 212-633-3820, and E-mail: reprints@elsevier.com.

Critical Care Nursing Clinics of North America is covered in *MEDLINE/PubMed (Index Medicus), International Nursing Index, Nursing Citation Index, Cumulative Index to Nursing and Allied Health Literature, and RNdex Top 100.*

Contributors

CONSULTING EDITOR

JAN FOSTER, PhD, APRN, CNS
Formerly, Associate Professor, College of Nursing, Texas Woman's University, Houston; President, Nursing Inquiry and Intervention, Inc, The Woodlands, Texas

EDITOR

JAN FOSTER, PhD, APRN, CNS
Formerly, Associate Professor, College of Nursing, Texas Woman's University, Houston; President, Nursing Inquiry and Intervention, Inc, The Woodlands, Texas

AUTHORS

MICHELE C. BALAS, PhD, RN, FCCM
Associate Professor, Center of Excellence in Critical and Complex Care, College of Nursing, The Ohio State University, Columbus, Ohio

KAREN BERGMAN, PhD, RN, CNRN
Bronson Hospital, Western Michigan University, Kalamazoo, Michigan

PATRICIA A. BLISSITT, PhD, RN, CCRN, CNRN, SCRN, CCNS, CCM, ACNS-BC
Neuroscience Clinical Nurse Specialist, Harborview Medical Center and Swedish Medical Center; Associate Professor, Clinical Faculty, University of Washington School of Nursing, Seattle, Washington

SCOTT B. DAVIDSON, MD, FACS
Trauma Surgery Services, Bronson Hospital, Kalamazoo, Michigan

KRISTEN DITCH, PharmD, BCPS
Clinical Pharmacy Specialist, Department of Pharmacy, Neuro-Trauma Burn Intensive Care Unit, UMass Memorial Medical Center, Worcester, Massachusetts

NATALIE A. DUMONT, BS
Research Assistant, Department of Nursing Science, College of Nursing, University of Arkansas for Medical Sciences, Little Rock, Arkansas

JAN FOSTER, PhD, APRN, CNS
Formerly, Associate Professor, College of Nursing, Texas Woman's University, Houston; President, Nursing Inquiry and Intervention, Inc, The Woodlands, Texas

KEVIN FRANKLIN, BS, CFRN
West Michigan Air Care, Kalamazoo, Michigan

CARMELO GRAFFAGNINO, MD, FNCS
Professor, Department of Neurology, Duke University, Durham, North Carolina

DAWN JOHNSTON, BSN, BA, CFRN
West Michigan Air Care, Kalamazoo, Michigan

ROBERTA KAPLOW, PhD, APRN-CCNS, AOCNS, CCRN
Clinical Nurse Specialist, Emory University Hospital, Atlanta, Georgia

ANNA KRUPP, MS, RN
Clinical Nurse Specialist, Department of Nursing and Patient Care Services, University of Wisconsin Hospital and Clinics, Madison, Wisconsin

SIMON LEUNG, MS, PharmD, BCPS
Department of Pharmacy, Memorial Regional Hospital, Hollywood, Florida

ELLYN E. MATTHEWS, PhD, RN, AOCNS, CBSM, FAAN
Associate Professor; Elizabeth Stanley Cooper Endowed Chair in Oncology Nursing, Department of Nursing Science, College of Nursing, University of Arkansas for Medical Sciences, Little Rock, Arkansas

KRISTIN MEDEIROS, PharmD, BCPS
PGY2 Critical Care Pharmacy Resident, Department of Pharmacy, UMass Memorial Medical Center, Worcester, Massachusetts

MELISSA A. MILLER, PharmD, BCPS
Clinical Pharmacy Manager, Emergency Medicine, New York-Presbyterian Hospital, New York, New York

DAIWAI M. OLSON, PhD, RN, CCRN, FNCS
Associate Professor, Department of Neurology and Neurotherapeutics, University of Texas Southwestern, Dallas, Texas

KYLONI PHILLIPS, MSN, APRN, ACNP-BC, CNRN
Nurse Practitioner, Department of Neurology and Neurotherapeutics, University of Texas Southwestern, Dallas, Texas

PAUL RIGBY, BSN, CFRN
West Michigan Air Care, Kalamazoo, Michigan

GINA RIGGI, PharmD, BCPS, BCCCP
Department of Pharmacy, Jackson Memorial Hospital, Miami, Florida

BRIAN S. SMITH, PharmD
Director, Specialty Pharmacy Services, UMass Memorial Shields Pharmacy, Worcester, Massachusetts

DEBRA SULLIVAN, PhD, MSN, RN, CNE, COI
Core Faculty, School of Nursing MSN Program, School of Nursing Graduate Program, College of Health Sciences, Walden University, Minneapolis, Minnesota

J. MARK TANNER, DNP, RN
Clinical Instructor; Interim BSN Director, Department of Nursing Science, College of Nursing, University of Arkansas for Medical Sciences, Little Rock, Arkansas

CHRISTOPHER A. WEATHERSPOON, APRN, MS, FNP-BC
School of Nursing Graduate Program, Contributing Faculty, College of Health Sciences, Walden University, Minneapolis, Minnesota; Family Nurse Practitioner, Veteran Affairs, Tennessee Valley Health System, Fort Campbell, Kentucky

DEBORAH WEATHERSPOON, PhD, MSN, RN, CRNA
Core Faculty Leadership and Management Specialty, School of Nursing Graduate Program, College of Health Sciences, Walden University, Minneapolis, Minnesota

DINESH YOGARATNAM, PharmD, BCPS, BCCCP
Assistant Professor, Department of Pharmacy Practice, Massachusetts College of Pharmacy and Health Sciences University, Worcester, Massachusetts

ANTONIA ZAPANTIS, MS, PharmD, BCPS
Department of Pharmacy, Delray Medical Center, Delray Beach, Florida

Contents

psychiatric, and cognitive complications of oversedation, and multiple research-based strategies that minimize complications.

Application of Clinical Practice Guidelines for Pain, Agitation, and Delirium **241**

Anna Krupp and Michele C. Balas

Critically ill patients experience several severe, distressing, and often life-altering symptoms during their intensive care unit stay. A clinical practice guideline released by the American College of Critical Care Medicine provides a template for improving the care and outcomes of the critically ill through evidence-based pain, agitation, and delirium assessment, prevention, and management. Key strategies include the use of valid and reliable assessment tools, setting a desired sedation level target, a focus on light sedation, choosing appropriate sedative medications, the use of nonpharmacologic symptom management strategies, and engaging and empowering patients and their family to play an active role in their intensive care unit care.

Sleep Disturbances in Acutely Ill Patients with Cancer **253**

Ellyn E. Matthews, J. Mark Tanner, and Natalie A. Dumont

Intensive care units may place acutely ill patients with cancer at additional risk for sleep loss and associated negative effects. Research suggests that communication about sleep in patients with cancer is suboptimal and sleep problems are not regularly assessed or adequately treated throughout the cancer trajectory. However, many sleep problems and fatigue can be managed effectively. This article synthesizes the current literature regarding the prevalence, cause, and risk factors that contribute to sleep disturbance in the context of acute cancer care. It describes the consequences of poor sleep and discusses appropriate assessment and treatment options.

CRITICAL CARE NURSING CLINICS OF NORTH AMERICA

FORTHCOMING ISSUES

September 2016
Cardiac Arrhythmias
Mary G. Carey, *Editor*

December 2016
Mechanical Ventilation in the Critically Ill Patient: International Nursing Perspectives
Sandra Goldsworthy, *Editor*

March 2017
Infection in the Intensive Care Unit
Todd Tartavoulle and Jennifer Manning, *Editors*

RECENT ISSUES

March 2016
Neuromonitoring and Assessment
Catherine Harris, *Editor*

December 2015
Heart Failure
Jennifer Kitchens and Lenora Maze, *Editors*

September 2015
Palliative Care in Critical Care
Tonja M. Hartjes, *Editor*

Preface
An Update on Sleep and Sedation Issues in Critical Care

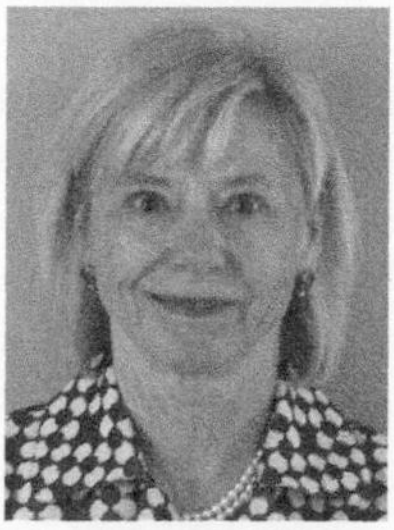

Jan Foster, PhD, APRN, CNS
Editor

More than a decade has passed since the first *Critical Care Nursing Clinics of North America* issue on sleep and sedation concerns experienced by critically ill patients was published. Much progress has been made in a relatively short time span. One thing that has not changed is the challenge of administering adequate sedation and analgesia during transportation of critically ill patients, both intrahospital and interfacility. Johnston and colleagues propose recommendations for selection, dosing, and timing of administration of sedatives and analgesics to optimize comfort and safety during and immediately following transport. Riggi, Zapantis, and Leung describe tolerance to sedatives, which can lead to excessive dosing, along with the risk for iatrogenic withdrawal. Both phenomena contribute to additional complications of sedative use. Recognition and prevention strategies are offered. Kaplow addresses sleep disturbances and interference with healing mechanisms in the critically ill, with a discussion of physiologic processes disrupted by environmental factors, patient factors, medications, and other aspects of patient management. The pharmacokinetics and pharmacodynamics of sedatives and analgesics used in critical illness are detailed by Yogaratnam and colleagues, with emphasis on tailoring drug regimens for patients with compromised renal and/or hepatic function to prevent adverse events. Blissitt addresses the physiologic consequences of mechanical ventilation on sleep and provides a menu of ventilator modes available to mitigate some of the problems. Standard sedation assessment methods in neuro-injured patients can be counter to management approaches that include minimal stimulation; also sedation can mask decreasing neurologic response patterns. Olson, Phillips, and Graffagnino offer alternative technological methods to augment traditional assessment techniques. Obstructive sleep apnea, often undiagnosed when patients enter the ICU, increases the risk of sedative use. Weatherspoon, Sullivan, and Weatherspoon describe screening tools and guidelines for sedation administration in this patient population. Foster discusses immediate and long-term complications of sedation, using the new

Crit Care Nurs Clin N Am 28 (2016) xi–xii
http://dx.doi.org/10.1016/j.cnc.2016.03.001 ccnursing.theclinics.com
0899-5885/16/$ – see front matter © 2016 Published by Elsevier Inc.

framework, post-ICU syndrome. A major advance over the past decade is the development of the Clinical Practice Guidelines for Pain, Agitation, and Delirium, described by Krupp and Balas in this issue, who bring the Guidelines to life with strategies for clinical application. Acutely ill patients with cancer experience unique sleep disruption patterns due to tumor pathophysiology, treatment modalities, symptomatology, psychosocial alterations, and comorbid medical conditions, explained by Matthews, Tanner, and Dumont. Methods of sleep assessment and interventions to promote sleep are described.

We hope that this update on sleep and sedation increases awareness of the potential for problems during critical illness beyond the disease or primary condition necessitating ICU care. The authors for each article have updated a review of the literature and incorporated the most current evidence; it is our intent that critical care professionals find practical application of this state of the science content on sleep and sedation issues for critically ill patients.

Jan Foster, PhD, APRN, CNS
Nursing Inquiry and Intervention, Inc
The Woodlands, TX 77381, USA

E-mail address:
jgwfoster@comcast.net

Sedation and Analgesia in Transportation of Acutely and Critically Ill Patients

Dawn Johnston, BSN, BA, CFRN[a,*], Kevin Franklin, BS, CFRN[a],
Paul Rigby, BSN, CFRN[a], Karen Bergman, PhD, RN, CNRN[b],
Scott B. Davidson, MD[c]

KEYWORDS

• Sedation • Analgesia • Transport • Intensive care • Guidelines • Critical care • Agitation • Pain

KEY POINTS

- Maintaining adequate sedation and analgesia in critically ill patients throughout transport poses unique challenges and potential threats to patient and provider safety, requiring coordination, planning, and forethought.
- Selection and dosing of sedation and analgesia should be based on situation and patient conditions and ideally titrated to effective response without adversely affecting vital signs (VSs).
- Use of sedation and analgesia scoring is recommended as an objective tool to achieve more consistent levels of therapeutic sedation and analgesia.
- Development and implementation of regional clinical practice guidelines would be helpful to maintain consistent sedation/analgesia and patient safety throughout transport.

INTRODUCTION

Sedation and analgesia for critically ill patients should not be unnecessarily interrupted during transport; however, many variables, such as patient instability and inadequate provider training, may increase the risk for this occurrence.[1] Evidence-based research toward best practices is scarce in this subject area, leaving health care providers to extrapolate primarily from recommendations intended for the ICU. Some of the more helpful recent developments are proposed clinical practice guidelines and

This article is an update of an article previously published in *Critical Care Nursing Clinics of North America*, Volume 17, Issue 3, September 2005.
The authors have nothing to disclose and no conflicts of interest.

[a] West Michigan Air Care, PO Box 50406, Kalamazoo, MI 49005, USA; [b] Bronson Hospital, Western Michigan University, 601 John Street, Box 88, Kalamazoo, MI 49007, USA; [c] Trauma Surgery Services, Bronson Hospital, 601 John Street, Kalamazoo, MI 49007, USA
* Corresponding author.
E-mail address: dmjohnston@aircare.org

Crit Care Nurs Clin N Am 28 (2016) 137–154
http://dx.doi.org/10.1016/j.cnc.2016.02.004 ccnursing.theclinics.com

checklists for planning and documentation of patient condition while off the unit for procedures.[2,3] Although this is a step in the right direction, best practice recommendations are still needed to guide both in-hospital and out-of-hospital transports of critically ill patients currently managed with medication as needed, restraint orders, and limited manpower and resources.

Appropriately medicated ICU patients benefit via reduced myocardial oxygen demand, decreased work of breathing, and reduced metabolic and hormonal responses to acute and critical illness.[4] Pursuit of optimal sedation and analgesia in transport is necessary to assure there are no gaps in the integrated, interdisciplinary approach currently recommended to provide physical and psychological comfort to critically ill patients to improve outcomes.[5,6]

Case review

A 68-year-old male patient in cardiac arrest was resuscitated at a small community hospital and transfer was arranged to a facility with interventional cardiac catheterization laboratory and critical care services. According to staff, the patient was combative after resuscitation and given 2 mg of lorazepam (Ativan) and 50-μg and 100-μg doses of fentanyl (Sublimaze) with little change neurologically. Intubation became necessary for airway protection. On the flight team's arrival, the second intubation attempt was in progress. Neuromuscular blockers (NMBs) given prior to intubation included 2 doses of succinylcholine (Anectine) and a single dose of vecuronium (Norcuron). Sedation had not been given recently and the patient's VSs were now blood pressure (BP) 190/120 mm Hg, heart rate (HR) 105 beats per minute, and oxygen saturations 86% with assisted ventilations. Additional sedation was provided by the transport team, including the recommended intubating dose of ketamine (Ketalar) at 1.5 mg/kg. The team successfully intubated the patient; however, he developed postsedation hypotension, requiring additional fluids and a vasopressor to keep BP above 90 mm Hg during transport.

This vignette highlights several important points in the management of sedation and analgesia (pain control) in transport:

- First, adequate sedation and analgesia must be in effect during uncomfortable procedures, such as intubation. These needs are not met by NMBs (paralytics) like succinylcholine (Anectine) and vecuronium (Norcuron).
- Second, nursing staff should be aware of onset and duration of the sedatives and analgesics administered and assess for signs of returning awareness and pain (ie, hypertension and tachycardia). In this case, the patient's BP indicated awareness, anxiety, and/or pain that he could not express because of the paralytic agents in his system.
- Individual response to sedation/analgesia may vary depending on many factors, including cardiac output, chronic tolerance, liver and kidney dysfunction, and drug-drug interactions. The addition of a single dose of ketamine provided both sedation and pain control, a double benefit unique to ketamine. This patient developed hypotension, an unusual occurrence in the use of ketamine for normotensive or hypertensive patients. Ketamine dosing was subsequently found to require scaled decreases in states of lower perfusion, such as cardiogenic shock and hypovolemic shock, and protocols were appropriately changed.[7,8] This recommendation is similar to other sedation/analgesia agents, most of which require decreased dosing in low perfusion states.[1]

This article describes common challenges in keeping critically ill patients sedated and treated for pain during various phases of transport. Care is taken to emphasize the difference between sedatives, analgesics, and NMBs, the latter frequently mistaken for sedation. Discussion of the most frequently used agents includes a focus on transport-related concerns, such as onset, duration, and hemodynamic profile. Explanations of concerns relating to sedation and analgesia throughout interfacility transport are discussed along with shorter in-hospital transfers, such as transfers to testing or to another unit. Tools frequently used for assessing the effectiveness of sedation and analgesia in transport are reviewed and discussed, and clinical practice guidelines are reviewed.

IN-HOSPITAL VERSUS OUT-OF-HOSPITAL SEDATION AND ANALGESIA IN TRANSPORT

Keeping critically ill patients comfortable and adequately sedated in a hospital setting can be challenging for an ICU nurse, and the need for these medications increases during transport to keep patients calm and compliant.[4] Transferring a critically ill patient to a different facility or to a different area within a facility requires careful preparation, monitoring, and cooperation between caregivers to assure the maintenance of optimum sedation, analgesia, and patient safety. Movement is frequently painful for the patient and contributes to a more wakeful state. Additional stimulation factors encountered in the average transport, whether by ground or air, include noise, vibration, and changes in temperature.[2,9] Patients vary in their acuity, pain tolerance, and need for sedation, complicated by the conditions of transport, which create stimuli that lead to increased pain and wakefulness. Patients tolerate movement better when sedated and preemptively treated for pain; therefore, premedication for transport is advised.[5] Careful attention to VSs is necessary to ensure that no adverse effects, such as hypoxia and hypotension, are encountered.[1] Intubated patients in general prefer not to be awake or remember the experience because there is almost always discomfort associated with the presence of an indwelling endotracheal (ET) tube.[10] Even wakeful, nonintubated ICU patients likely tolerate transfers better when medicated beforehand. In-hospital transfers tend to be shorter events compared with out-of-hospital transfers, but both types of transfers are discussed due to their similarities.

SEDATION AND ANALGESIA DIFFERENCES

Nurses and other health care professionals must keep in mind the different pharmacologic properties of various sedation, analgesic, and NMB agents. Although commonly used together, it is important to understand the dosing and expected duration of action of each so that patients are not undermedicated or overmedicated. All patients should be monitored for hypotension, the need for stabilizing measures, and, possibly, drug reversal.[11,12]

Sedation

Most agents used as sedatives provide sedation only, not analgesia. The level of sedation is dose dependent, providing anxiety relief, relaxation, and varying levels of depressed consciousness. It can be difficult to predict how a patient will respond to sedatives, so nonintubated patients should be monitored for the need for airway assistance.[12]

Analgesia (Pain Control)

Drugs classified as analgesics provide pain control and often have a small sedative effect that is dose dependent. Pain control is necessary to prevent a cascade of negative physical and psychological effects as well as facilitating genuine rest periods that promote healing.[5]

Neuromuscular Blockers

NMBs provide neither sedation nor analgesia but relax all muscles, including the diaphragm. NMBs are sometimes required for intubation or to achieve ventilator tolerance, especially during transport. Despite appropriate dosing of sedation and analgesia, sometimes NMBs are required to achieve ventilator synchrony or safety in transport.[4]

Fig. 1 distinguishes the difference between common agents used in the emergency department and ICU for sedation, analgesia, and NMB.

CHALLENGES OF CRITICALLY ILL, UNSTABLE PATIENTS IN TRANSPORT

Risk of Injury to Patient and Personnel

Transferring patients puts both patients and providers at increased risk for adverse events.[3,9,13] Providers must protect patients by keeping track of multiple pieces of equipment attached to the patient and avoiding dislodgement of IVs, ET tubes, and other devices. During transfers, adequate sedation and analgesia can mitigate these risks by keeping the patient calm and compliant as well as comfortable.[4] All patients should be assessed for risk to themselves and the health care providers, especially in cases of air transport. Acutely ill psychiatric patients or prisoners, for example, may present with unpredictable behavior. There are noted cases of patients attempting to injure pilots or crew during transport, and at times injuring themselves, so careful assessment of the need for sedation prior to and during transport is critical.[14]

Timing Sedation and Analgesia to Prevent Pain with Movement

Administration should be guided by current and anticipated needs of the patient.[5] Therefore, sedatives and analgesics are often provided prior to movement with knowledge of onset time. For example, IV midazolam takes only 2 minutes to 5 minutes for effect, whereas IV lorazepam has a 15-minute to 20-minute onset time.[5] Distinctions such as these become important when a combative patient requires immediate restraint.

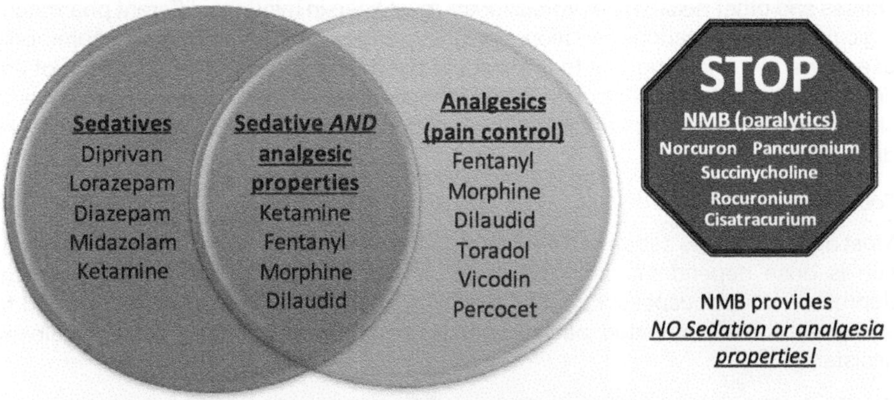

Fig. 1. These medications are generally classified as either sedation or analgesia based on their primary effects. Some can provide both, but the secondary effect tends to be mild. NMBs, in contrast, provide no sedation or analgesia but only paralyze a patient's muscles, including those required for breathing. In addition to ventilator support, patients given NMBs require sedation and analgesia for ET tube tolerance.

Potential for Hypotension

In unstable patients, it should be remembered that most IV sedatives and analgesics can lower BP depending on the dose and patient condition.[1] One solution to this dilemma may be to alternate drugs throughout the transport. For example, analgesia can be given just prior to transport and sedation given 15 minutes later when the greatest potential for hypotension from the analgesia has passed, as demonstrated by VSs. Another approach may be to obtain an order for additional IV fluids as necessary to treat hypotension during transport, but this assumes no fluid overload concerns exist. Ideally, patients are adequately pain controlled first, followed by just enough sedation, with hemodynamic stability maintained during transport.[5]

Nonintubated Patients

Many acute and critically ill patients are not intubated. In nonintubated patients, sedation and analgesia should be titrated to an effective dose that minimizes side effects on oxygenation and VSs.[1,12] Sometimes, however, a patient's status is so tenuous that sedation/analgesia must wait because other life threats take precedence. Administering sedation and analgesia to make a patient comfortable when unstable is risky. Transport crews should be skilled at identifying patients' needs for oxygenation and/or BP support and select the appropriate interventions while meeting sedation and analgesia needs only with respect to the patient's condition. When impending airway failure and hypotension occur together, this requires an attempt to optimize the patient's BP with appropriate IV fluids, blood products, or vasopressors before administering rapid sequence induction drugs that can lower BP even further and lead to cardiac arrest.[15] Transport crews must be prepared to manage unstable patients with full knowledge of the effects of the sedation and analgesia they have access to, sometimes avoiding them entirely until the patient is stable enough to tolerate them.

Special Patient Populations

Acute and critically ill patients with painful conditions almost universally require analgesia (using an appropriate pain scale), and this intervention should be given before sedation, so less sedation is required.[6] Some conditions require special considerations:

- Liver and kidney dysfunction may reduce the dosage or frequency of administration, depending on how a drug is metabolized. Hepatic or renal clearance of many drugs may be slowed in these patients.[4] VS monitoring and pain and sedation scoring should be used to help the transport team identify reduced sedation and analgesia needs (see sedation and analgesia tables).
- Head-injured patients, in particular, cannot afford even 1 episode of hypotension or hypoxia, which has been shown to adversely affect neurologic outcomes. This patient population requires cautious but adequate administration of sedatives and analgesics.[16]

Level of Training

A different but real safety concern is providers' level of training. They should be experienced with critical care patients, preferably certified for critical care transport, and proficient with sedation/analgesia drugs by IV push and by infusion. Programmable pumps can assist with precise dosing and attending personnel should be well trained on this equipment to titrate infusions to therapeutic effect.[9,17,18]

PROVIDING SEDATION AND ANALGESIA DURING INTERFACILITY TRANSPORT

Sedative Selection and Dosing

Pain should be treated preemptively before potentially painful procedures.[5] For many patients, this includes movement from a bed to transport stretcher and vibrations while riding on a gurney. Whether intubated or not, it is recommended to treat pain effectively in critically ill patients by monitoring VSs and using a valid and reliable pain scale tool, such as the Critical-Care Pain Observation Tool (CPOT) before administering sedation. This is called *analgesia-first sedation*.[5] Once pain is controlled, a light level of sedation is preferred in the ICU using a valid and reliable sedation scale, such as the Richmond Agitation-Sedation Scale (RASS), to produce shorter durations of mechanical ventilation and to shorten ICU length of stay.[5] These same goals can be established for transport as well; however, because transport is essentially a painful procedure, patients likely require increases in analgesia and sedation to tolerate movement.[4] Using the least amount for the desired effect is ideal, but context matters. Occasionally, a rapid-onset sedative is the first-line drug of choice to prevent an agitated patient from causing adverse events, but this is the exception. When selecting as-needed sedatives and analgesics, adhere to the following recommendations, carefully monitoring for adverse responses:

1. Treat pain effectively first while monitoring VS and CPOT.[5]
2. Add light sedation and increase only as required, while monitoring VS and RASS.[5]
3. Treat pain preemptively, before painful procedures (like movement).[5]
4. Use IV opioids first line for non-neuropathic pain. Add oral gabapentin or carbamazepine for neuropathic pain.[5]
5. Use nonopioid analgesics to decrease amount of opioids required (and therefore adverse effects like hypotension).[5]
6. A nonbenzodiazepine, such as propofol or dexmedetomidine, is preferred for sedation. These have so far been superior to benzodiazepines when comparing length of ventilator therapy and outcomes for ICU-ventilated patients.[5]

Tables 1 and **2** provide a quick practical reference for commonly used analgesics and sedatives in the ICU and in transport.

Phase I: Preparing the Patient for Transport

A patient with multitrauma had just been intubated by the ER physician when the transport team arrived. The staff reported sedation had been given during the intubation and the team reconfirmed ET placement. During preparations for transport, the intubated patient began moving his arms and tried to sit up in bed. He was quickly restrained and resedated. Hospital staff clarified that etomidate was given prior, a procedural anesthetic with a short half-life of approximately 5 minutes.

Transport teams can set themselves up for success or failure during this initial phase of transport. Speed is less desirable than is stabilization before transport, although complete stabilization likely needs to be accomplished by the receiving facility.[9] A good plan requires being familiar with a patient's medication status, including sedation and analgesia needs and responses prior to in-hospital or out-of-hospital transfer.[9] Although physical restraints in the hospital are an acceptable safety net to prevent falls or accidental removal of devices, such as IVs and ET tubes, these are generally not relied on in the air transport environment, so adequate pharmacologic restraint is important for safety as well as for meeting patients' comfort needs.[19]

Inadequacies during transfer of care can lead to a disorganized, uninformed transport crew and predispose patients to adverse events.[9] Logically, efficient transfer of care to the transport team usually requires the assistance of the sending registered nurse (RN) at the bedside to provide report and answer questions. It is also a safe practice to discontinue, cap, or drain current therapies and those no longer in use, such as dialysis, gastric drainage, ET suctioning, and all infusion lines that are nonessential. Reporting the sedation/analgesia history to the crew, including times and doses of administration, helps them develop a sedation/analgesia plan for transport. Helpful information to provide to the crew includes drugs, dosage, and average sedation and pain scoring, if known. The transport crew should also be made aware of drug allergies, which may include sedatives or analgesics they may have been planning to use from their protocols. After formulating a plan for sedation and analgesia, the transport team should have unit doses prepared for quick retrieval and administration. Following these simple steps will produce a well-coordinated, multidisciplinary approach, which is recommended for safe and uninterrupted sedation and analgesia.[6]

Although sedative and analgesic infusions can provide the most consistent and hassle-free maintenance of sedation/analgesia in transport, the need to use a limited number of transport pumps for other essential infusions, such as vasopressors and antibiotics, may make an IV push method necessary. As the patient is prepared for transport, it is important that this IV push line or saline lock be readily identifiable and accessible. Entanglements can be avoided by simplifying infusion therapy wherever possible, for example, completing and discontinuing IV lines and piggyback extensions no longer in use. Because glass bottles are avoided, the transport team may draw up propofol (Diprivan) in a 30-mL syringe and attach to drip tubing for infusion pump as a safer option, to rule out potential breakage en route.[9]

It is advisable to medicate patients for pain before each move and before transport, as their conditions allow, just as before a painful procedure.[5] When a patient is prone to hypotension, sedation and analgesia should be scaled. As a rule, drugs should be administered over 2 minutes. Rapid administration can cause adverse side effects, such as a sudden drop in BP and/or nausea. Ideally patients are adequately medicated to an acceptable RASS or CPOT score before departure from the sending facility.[5,20,21]

Phase II: Sedation/Analgesia Within the Transport

The intubated patient was given morphine (5 mg) for pain and light sedation by the sending nurse and monitored for response before sedation was given. He became sedate and his BP dropped to 82/35 mm Hg and recovered to baseline normal within 5 to 10 minutes. As the crew departed with the patient, fentanyl was administered to treat pain but dosing was decreased to prevent a recurrence of the observed hypotension to analgesia. The patient became more active and low-dose ketamine was also administered for sedation and pain control. Just prior to administration, the patient's movement caused tension on cables and lines, pulling off 2 monitor leads. These were replaced and additional analgesia was given for presumed pain, but the IV had unknowingly become dislodged. VSs remained stable and the patient continued to become increasingly active until the dislodged IV was discovered.

IVs should be well secured with tape to avoid dislodgement, but an active patient may defeat a transport team's best efforts. The unpredictability of active intubated patients presents a risk to themselves and personnel.[9] A squirming patient is at an increased risk of falling when moved. During an average transfer, a patient is moved 2 to 6 times, depending on the configuration and necessary arrangements: to the transport team's cot, into the transfer vehicle, from the transfer vehicle, onto the receiving hospital bed, and so forth. Certain situations can warrant additional transfers, for example, if a ground run to or from the airport is necessary.[9] All these moves

Table 1
Analgesics

Analgesics	Onset	Duration	Dosage	Excretion/Metabolism	Common Side Effects
(IV) morphine sulfate (morphine)	IV: 15–30 min Peak 30–60 min	IV: ~ 1.5–4 h	IV: 0.05–0.1 mg/kg	Hepatic glucuronidation Excretion: urine 12%, feces 10% Half-life 1.5–4.5 h	CNS depression, flushing, hypotension (with rapid administration), nausea/vomiting (with rapid administration), respiratory depression (larger dosages and/or rapid administration), constipation
(PO) morphine sulfate (morphine)	PO: 60 min	PO: 4–5 h	PO: 15–30 mg Q 4 h	Hepatic glucuronidation Excretion: urine 12%, feces 10% Half-life 1.5–4.5 h	CNS depression, constipation, nausea/vomiting (less common then IV), respiratory depression (larger dosages), hypotension (larger dosages)
Fentanyl (Sublimaze)	IV: 1–3 min; peak 5 min	IV: 30–60 min	IV: 0.5–2 μg/kg	Hepatically metabolized Excretion: urine 75% Half-life 2–4 h	Dysphoria, nasal itching, nausea/vomiting (with rapid administration), hypotension (with rapid administration), respiratory depression (larger dosages and/or rapid administration), chest wall rigidity (uncommon except in high dosages with rapid administration)
Sufentanil (Sufenta)	IV: 1–3 min Peak 5 min	Dose dependent	IV: 1–8 μg/kg	Hepatically metabolized Excretion: urine Half-life 2–6 h (dose dependent)	Respiratory depression (larger dosages), bradycardia, chest wall rigidity (uncommon except in high dosages with rapid administration)

Hydromorphone (Dilaudid)	IV: 15–30 min Peak: 30–90 min	IV: 4–5 h	IV: 0.2–1 mg q 2–3 h	Hepatically metabolized Excretion: urine	Respiratory depression (larger dosages and/or rapid administration), hypotension (larger dosages and/or rapid administration), nausea/vomiting, flushing, dysphoria
(IV) methadone hydrochloride (methadone)	IV: 5–10 min Peak: 15–20 min	IV: 4–6 h	IV: 2.5–10 mg q 8–12 h	Hepatically metabolized Excretion: urine	Respiratory depression (larger dosages), hypotension (larger dosages), nausea/vomiting
(PO) methadone hydrochloride (methadone)	PO: 30–60 min Peak: 30–60 min	PO: 6–8 h	PO: 5–20 mg q 8–12 h	Hepatically metabolized Excretion: urine	Respiratory depression (larger dosages), hypotension (larger dosages), nausea/vomiting (less common then IV)
Acetaminophen/codeine phosphate (Tylenol with Codeine)	PO: 30–60 min Peak: 60–90 min	PO: 4–6 h	PO: 15 mg/300 mg–60 mg/1000 mg (codeine/acetaminophen)	Hepatic glucuronidation Hepatically metabolized Excretion: urine	Liver failure (with high daily dosing or underlying liver disease), nausea/vomiting, drowsiness, respiratory depression (larger dosages)
Ketorolac tromethamine (Toradol)	IV: 1–3 min	IV: 4–6 h	IV: 15–30 mg q 6 h	Hepatically metabolized Excretion: urine	headache, nausea/vomiting, abdominal pain
Gabapentin (Neurontin)	PO: 2–3 h	PO: 5–7 h	PO: 300–900 mg tid (must start qd and increase slowly)	Limited metabolism Excretion: urine	somnolence, ataxia, fatigue

Data from Refs.[25–41]

Table 2
Sedatives

Sedatives	Onset	Duration	Dosage	Excretion/Metabolism	Common Side Effects
Alprazolam (Xanax)	PO: 1–2 h (time to peak)	PO: ~4 h	PO: 0.25–0.5 mg TID	Hepatically metabolized Excretion: urine Half-life 11 h	CNS depression, anterograde amnesia
Dexmedetomidine (Precedex)	IV: 5–10 min	IV: 1–2 h	IV load: 1 μg/kg over 10 min IV drip: 0.2–0.7 μg/kg/h	Hepatically mbolized Excretion: urine Half-life: 6–60 min	Bradycardia, hypotension
Propofol (Diprivan)	IV: 30 s	IV: 3–10 min	IV drip: 5–50 μg/kg/min	Hepatically metabolized Half-life 40 min	hypotension, respiratory depression, bradycardia (pediatrics)
Haloperidol (Haldol)	IV: ~5 min IM: 20–30 min	IV: ~4 h IM: 4–8 h	IV: 0.5–10 mg q 30 min IV drip: 0.5–2 mg/h IM: 2.5–10 mg	Hepatically metabolized Excretion: urine Half-life: 21–24 h	Prolonged QT syndrome, extrapyramidal symptoms, anticholinergic effects
Ketamine (Ketalar)	IV: 30 s IM: 3–4 min	IV: 5–10 min IM: 12–25 min	IV: 0.2–1.0 mg/kg IM: 2–4 mg/kg	Hepatically metabolized Half-life 10–15 min No dose adjustments required	Airway complications, respiratory depression, hallucinations/delirium
Lorazepam (Ativan)	IV: 1–3 min IM: 15–20 min	IV: ~6–8 h IM: ~ 6–8 h	IV: 0.02–0.04 mg/kg IV drip: 0.01–0.1 mg/kg/h IM: 0.05 mg/kg PO: 2–6 mg daily in divided doses	Hepatically metabolized Excretion: urine Half-life ~14–18 h Use caution in patients with renal and hepatic impairment	CNS depression, paradoxic reactions (delirium)
Midazolam (Versed)	IV: 3–5 min IM: ~15 min	IV: <2 h (dose dependent) IM: up to 6 h	IV: 0.01–0.05 mg/kg IV drip: 0.02–0.1 mg/kg/h	Hepatically metabolized Excretion: urine Half-life 2–7 h Use caution with severe hepatic impairment	Hypotension, respiratory depression, CNS depression
Quetiapine (Seroquel)	PO: 1.5 h (time to peak)	PO: 8–12 h	PO: 50 mg BID (max 400 mg daily)	Hepatically metabolized Excretion: urine Half-life: ~6–7 h	Prolonged QT syndrome, CNS depression

Abbreviations: CNS, central nervous system; IM, intramuscular; max, maximum.
Data from Refs.[5,41–50]

present potential obstacles to ongoing sedation and analgesia if a patient breaks though the medication. This is most likely with a sedative like propofol (Diprivan), in which patients tend to sleep soundly until stimulated. Having alternative options on-hand, such as IV push sedation and analgesia, is helpful in making these moves comfortable and safe for the patient and providers.[11] Breakthrough awareness during sedation efforts is a good reason transporting personnel should know the onset and duration of sedation and analgesia. This knowledge can limit the damage done by a suddenly combative patient reaching for the IV or ET tube.

Maintaining adequate perfusion and VSs in transport is a priority and these may be adversely affected by liberal use of sedation and analgesia. Keep in mind the patient's hemodynamic tolerance for medications and pace drugs appropriately.[11] Evidence exists for lightening of sedation whenever possible for ICU patients to prevent delirium and other negative effects of long-term sedation and analgesia, but this is not practical in the transport setting where safety demands take precedence. Stimulation exaggerates the need for appropriate sedation and analgesia and patients often require higher doses than when in a stationary ICU bed.[11] In general, the transport crew medicates to avoid undersedation and inadequate pain control while maintaining hemodynamics.

Phase III: Completing the Transport/Receiving the Patient from the Transport Team

The dislodged IV was replaced. Despite receiving appropriate doses of sedation and analgesia during transport, the patient generated repeated ventilator alarms, coughing against the ET tube and prompting the team to provide NMB. On arrival, the receiving health care team helped transfer the patient to the bed and placed him on the monitor while medical staff received report. The receiving RN was not informed about the use of the NMB. A first BP cycled 5 minutes after arrival with the following VSs: BP 183/77 mm Hg, HR 128 beats per minute, respiratory rate 22, and PO 97%. The patient began to move and nearly self-extubated.

The receiving nurse needs key information, such as allergies, stability of the patient, and dosages and response to medication during transport. Ideally, the receiving nurse has a sedation/analgesia plan (and orders) in case these are needed as soon as the patient arrives. The first action after moving the patient to the hospital bed should be to obtain VSs to establish level of stability. If a patient arrives combative or in some other state of emergency, however, these threats should take first priority.

When receiving report from the transport team, the receiving nurse should be alert to the selection, dosing, and timing of sedation/analgesia/NMB administration, which may now be different from what was used at the sending facility. Coordinating the final transfer to the receiving unit safely involves a successful transition of infusions from transport pumps to unit pumps with no lapses in pharmocotherapy. Sedated ICU patients should experience no lags in medication that inadvertently increase pain or awareness.[5]

Transport teams should anticipate needs at the receiving facility, such as keeping the patient still during delicate, time-dependent procedures.[4] For example, when transferring an intubated post–cardiac arrest patient to the cardiovascular laboratory, transport crews may use a long-acting paralytic if a patient is still moving and at risk of self-extubation despite adequate doses of sedation/analgesia.

Toward the Development of a Sedation/Analgesia Checklist

To date, there is no evidence-based clinical practice guideline that directs the sedation/analgesia management of critically ill patients during transport, although preliminary efforts are moving in this direction, with the most progress being made for general patient safety and logistics of intrahospital patient transport.[3] Ideally, any type of transport guideline should be finely tuned and validated by the group of health care professionals using it. The checklist in **Box 1** is a good starting point for managing sedation and analgesia through the 3 phases of transport.

PROVIDING SEDATION AND ANALGESIA DURING IN-HOSPITAL TRANSPORTS

When transports within the hospital are necessary, it is usually of short duration to inpatient testing or to transfer a patient to another unit. Increases in sedation and analgesia are often necessary to make these in-house transfers tolerable for a critically ill

Box 1
A suggested checklist to maintain appropriate sedation/analgesia for acute and critically ill patients throughout transport

Preparing for transport

- Obtain patient report, including medication allergies, sedation/analgesia/NMB administration history, and response.
- Assess patient, including airway needs and hemodynamic, renal, and hepatic tolerances.
- Obtain VS and baseline scoring for sedation (RASS) and analgesia (CPOT).
- Formulate sedation/analgesia plan for transport, preferably using analgesia-first sedation.
- Coordinate all relevant logistics:
  - IV sites working, secured
  - All unnecessary entanglement risks removed, such as unused IV tubing
  - Avoid glass infusion bottles in transport.
  - Have unit doses already drawn up, labeled, and alcohol swabs available for cleansing IV ports.
  - Mark push port before departure and keep positioned in a readily accessible location.
  - Avoid leaking narcotics. Keep caps (not needles) on the end of syringes.
- Medicate before movement and as needed after checking VS.
- Assure adequate lift assistance is present for gentle and controlled transfers.
- Evaluate success of plan through ongoing scoring and adjust accordingly.

In transport

- Keep labeled unit doses of sedation and analgesia readily accessible.
- Check VSs and assess pain/agitation before administration and titrate accordingly.
- Double-check IV sites during administration.
- Know onset and duration of sedation/analgesia.
- Enlist adequate assistance to assure every move/turn/transfer is gentle and well controlled.
- Continue to medicate before movement.
- Evaluate sedation and pain levels through ongoing scoring.

Completing the transport/receiving

- Assure adequate assistance is present for each patient move.
- Provide report, including medication allergies, sedation/analgesia/NMB administration, and response.
- Assist in obtaining VSs and assuring a smooth transition with no pauses in adequate sedation, analgesia, or patient safety.

patient.[4] This requires VS monitoring and as well as ensuring that the nurse has adequate supplies for medicating the patient as needed.[3]

Consider that pain, and therefore agitation, is likely to increase when moving patients and plan to medicate preemptively.[5] Know onset times for sedatives and analgesics and time them far enough in advance for peak effect during movement. Being aware of the duration and hemodynamic effects of these medications and correlating dosing to patient condition is, therefore, necessary.[10] In addition, wherever possible, the stimulation of a critically ill patient should be minimized while in transport.

Basic logistics are a concern even when moving patients a short distance. Assure there are no entanglement risks from IVs or other therapies or equipment, which can lead to interruptions in sedation/analgesia. Once movement begins, it can be difficult to keep IV lines from becoming tangled. This can create a potential delay in ongoing sedation/analgesia as the nurse sorts the lines for a push port. Seeking a

Table 3
Critical-Care Pain Observation Tool

Indicator	Description	Score	
Facial expression	No muscular tension observed	Relaxed, neutral	0
	Presence of frowning, brow lowering, orbit tightening, and levator contraction	Tense	*1*
	All of the above facial movements plus eyelid tightly closed	Grimacing	*2*
Body movements	Does not move at all (does not necessarily mean absence of pain)	Absence of movements	0
	Slow, cautious movements, touching or rubbing the pain site, seeking attention through movements	Protection	1
	Pulling tube, attempting to sit up, moving limbs/thrashing, not following commands, striking at staff, trying to climb out of bed	Restlessness	2
Muscle tension Evaluation by passive flexion and extension of upper extremities	No resistance to passive movements	Relaxed	*0*
	Resistance to passive movements	Tense, rigid	*1*
	Strong resistance to passive movements, inability to complete them	Very tense or rigid	*2*
Compliance with the ventilator (intubated patients)	Alarms not activated, easy ventilation	Tolerating ventilator or movement	*0*
	Alarms stop spontaneously	Coughing but tolerating	1
	Asynchrony: blocking ventilation, alarms frequently activated	Fighting ventilator	*2*
or			
Vocalization (extubated patients)	Talking in normal tone or no sound	Talking in normal tone or no sound	*0*
	Sighing, moaning	Sighing, moaning	*1*
	Crying out, sobbing	Crying out, sobbing	*2*
Total, range	Sum each category	—	0–8

Adapted from Gélinas C, Fillion L, Puntillo KA, et al. Validation of the critical-care pain observation tool in adult patients. Am J Crit Care 2006;15(4):420–7; and Gélinas C, Johnston C. Pain assessment in the critically ill ventilated adult: validation of the critical-care pain observation tool and physiologic indicators. Clin J Pain 2007;23(6):497–505.

guideline or checklist for transport can be a helpful tool in planning and organizing a patient transfer in the hospital.[3] Objective scoring like RASS and CPOT can be used when a patient is off the unit to guide sedation and analgesia.

OBJECTIVE SCORING SCALES

Studies show that pain in the ICU is not treated effectively in more than 50% of cases and this can hamper healing and even put patients at risk of PTSD.[5,22] Transfer clinicians need to use tools that reliably assess patients' need for sedation and analgesia throughout the transport process and the tools used for the ICU are an effective means for this.

Pain Scales

Two pain scales that have been well validated in intubated and nonintubated patients are the Behavioral Pain Scale and the CPOT.[5,21] These have been deemed reliable in most adult ICU patients who are unable to report pain. Exceptions include brain-injured patients and nonintubated patients unable to report pain.[5] Clinicians also need to discern when agitation-induced ventilator dyssynchrony requires analgesia and sedation verses conditions when ventilator alarms are not agitation-related, such as hiccups and seizures.[23] The CPOT tool is shown in **Table 3**.

Sedation Scales

Two valid and reliable sedation assessment tools for use in the ICU are the RASS and Sedation-Agitation Scale (SAS).[5,24] These scales measure the depth and quality of sedation. Ideally, light sedation should be provided when necessary and preferably after pain is addressed. This approach, along with avoiding benzodiazepines, has been shown to reduce total length of mechanical ventilation and shorten ICU length of stays.[5] Benzodiazepines may still be used, but research is beginning to show worse outcomes associated with their use.[5] The RASS tool is shown in **Table 4**, and the SAS tool is shown in **Table 5**.

Table 4
Richmond Agitation-Sedation Scale

Score	State	Description
+4	Combative	Overtly combative, violent, immediate danger to staff
+3	Very agitated	Pulls or removes tube(s) or catheter(s); aggressive
+2	Agitated	Frequent nonpurposeful movement, fights ventilator
+1	Restless	Anxious, but movements not aggressive or vigorous
0	Alert and calm	—
−1	Drowsy	Mot fully alert, but has sustained awakening (eye opening/eye contact) to *voice* (≥10 s)
−2	Light sedation	Briefly awakens with eye contact to *voice* (<10 s)
−3	Moderate sedation	Movement or eye opening to *voice* (but no eye contact)
−4	Deep sedation	No response to voice, but movement or eye opening to *physical* stimulation
−5	Unarousable	No response to voice or *physical* stimulation

Reprinted with permission of the American Thoracic Society. Copyright © 2015 American Thoracic Society. Sessler CN, Gosnell MS, Grap MJ, et al. The Richmond Agitation–Sedation Scale. American Journal of Respiratory and Critical Care Medicine 166(10):1338–44. The American Journal of Respiratory and Critical Care Medicine is an official journal of the American Thoracic Society.

Table 5
Riker Sedation-Agitation Scale

Score	Characteristic	Examples of Patients' Behavior
7	Dangerous agitation	Pulls at ET tube, tries to remove catheters, climbs over bed rail, strikes at staff, thrashes side to side
6	Very agitated	Does not calm despite frequent verbal reminding of limits, requires physical restraints, bites ET tube
5	Agitated	Is anxious or mildly agitated, attempts to sit up, calms down in response to verbal instructions
4	Calm and cooperative	Is calm, awakens easily, follows commands
3	Sedated	Is difficult to arouse, awakens to verbal stimuli or gentle shaking but drifts off again, follows simple commands
2	Very sedated	Arouses to physical stimuli but does not communicate or follow commands, may move spontaneously
1	Unarousable	Has minimal or no response to noxious stimuli, does not communicate or follow commands

From Riker R, Picard J, Frazer G. Prospective evaluation of the sedation-agitation scale for adult critically ill patients. Crit Care Med 1999;27:1326; with permission.

SUMMARY

When patients are transported in-hospital or out-of-hospital, they should not be uncomfortable or lack appropriate sedation when abundant pharmacologic options exist. They should also not fall into harm during the transfer due to undermedication or overmedication for their condition. Well-trained clinicians experienced in transport needs can provide appropriate sedation and analgesia to the patient based on ongoing assessments during a monitored transfer, preventing labile VSs and sentinel events. Preemptive sedation and analgesia before movement can prevent a spike in alertness or pain during transport. Acute and critically ill patients have a better opportunity for safe and comfortable transport if safe and effective sedation/analgesia is used.[4,5]

REFERENCES

1. Singh JM, MacDonald RD, Anghari M. Post-medication hypotension after administration of sedatives and opioids during critical care transport. Prehosp Emerg Care 2015;19:464–74.

2. Martin KA, Houp J. Ready-set-go! A clinical practice guideline that promotes safe care of the sedated patient before, during, and after transport. Poster Presentation at the American Association of Neuroscience Nurses (AANN) 46th Annual Educational Meeting. Anaheim, March 8–11, 2014.

3. Brunsveld-Reinders AH, Arbous MS, Kuiper SG, et al. A comprehensive method to develop a checklist to increase safety of intra-hospital transport of critically ill patients. Crit Care 2015;19:1–10.

4. Pollard B. Sedation, analgesia, and neuromuscular blockade. In: Granton J, McConachie I, Fuller J, editors. Handbook of ICU therapy. Cornwall (United Kingdom): Cambridge University Press; 2015. p. 187–96.

5. Barr J, Frazer GL, Puntillo K, et al. Clinical practice guidelines for the management of pain, agitation, and delirium in adult patients in the intensive care Unit. Crit Care Med 2013;41(1):263–306.
6. Barr J, Pandharipande PP. The pain, agitation, and delirium care Bundle: Synergistic benefits of implementing the 2013 pain, agitation, and delirium guidelines in an integrated and interdisciplinary Fashion. Crit Care Med 2013;41:114–23.
7. Waxman K, Shoemaker WC, Lippman M. Cardiovascular effects of anesthetic induction with Ketamine. Anesth Analg 1980;59:355–8.
8. Haas DA, Harper DG. Ketamine: a review of its pharmacologic properties and use in ambulatory anesthesia. Anesth Prog 1992;39:61–8.
9. Sethi D, Subramanian S. When place and time matter: how to conduct safe interhospital transfer of patients. Saudi J Anaesth 2014;8:104–13.
10. Schweickert WD, Kress JP. Strategies to optimize analgesia and sedation. Crit Care 2008;12(Supp 3):S6.
11. Tobias JD, Leder M. Procedural sedation: a review of sedative agents, monitoring, and management of complications. Saudi J Anaesth 2011;5:395–410.
12. Anesthesiologists, American Society for and Admin., Quality Mgt and Dept. Continuum of Depth of Sedation: Definition of General Anesthesia and Levels of Sedation/Analgesia. Approved by the ASA 1999 and last amended 2014.
13. Nelson A, Baptiste AS. Evidence-based practices for safe patient handling and movement. Online J Issues Nurs 2004;9:4.
14. Wheeler S, Wong B, L'Heureux R. Criteria for sedation of psychiatric patients for air transport in British Columbia. Br Columbia Med J 2009;51:346–9.
15. Sherren PB, Tricklebank S, Glover G. Development of a standard operating procedure and checklist for rapid sequence induction in the critically ill. Scand J Trauma Resusc Emerg Med 2014;22:41.
16. Bullock MR, Povlishock JT. Guidelines for the management of severe traumatic brain injury. J Neurotrauma 2007;24:S1–106.
17. National Highway Traffic Safety Administration. Guide for interfacility patient transfer. NHTSA proceedings, Alexandria, VA, 2003.
18. Commission on Accreditation of Medical Transport System, Approved 9th edition Accreditation Standards. Sandy Springs (SC): CAMTS; 2012.
19. Kupas DF, Wydro GC. Patient restraint in emergency medical Services systems. Prehosp Emerg Care 2002;6(3):340–5. National Association of EMS Physicians Position Paper.
20. Sessler CN, Gosnell MS, Grap MJ, et al. The Richmond agitation-sedation scale; validity and reliability in adult intensive care Unit patients. Am J Respir Crit Care Med 2002;166(10):1338–44.
21. Stites M. Observational pain scales in critically ill adults. Crit Care Nurse 2013; 33(3):68–77.
22. Ramnarain D, Gnirrip I, Schapendonk W. Poster presentation. Post-traumatic stress disorder after ICU discharge: results of a post-ICU aftercare program. Crit Care 2015;19:533.
23. Bambi S, Lucchini A, Manici M, et al. Pain assessment scales in nonverbal critically ill adult patients: ventilator-related issues. Crit Care Nurse 2014;34(1):14–5.
24. Wesley E, Truman B, Shintani A, et al. Monitoring sedation status over time in ICU patients: reliability and validity of the Richmond agitation-sedation scale (RASS). J Am Med Assoc 2003;289(22):2983–91.
25. Shir Y, Rosen G, Zeldin A, et al. Methadone is safe for treating hospitalized patients with severe pain. Can J Anaesth 2001;48(11):1109–13.

26. Maciejewski D. Sufentanil in anaesthesiology and intensive therapy [review]. Anaesthesiol Intensive Ther 2012;44(1):35–41.
27. Jeleazcov C, Saari TI, Ihmsen H, et al. Changes in total and unbound concentrations of sufentanil during target controlled infusion for cardiac surgery with cardiopulmonary bypass. Br J Anaesth 2012;109(5):698–706.
28. Melson TI, Boyer DL, Minkowitz HS, et al. Sufentanil sublingual tablet system vs. intravenous patient-controlled analgesia with morphine for postoperative pain control: a randomized, active-comparator trial. Pain Pract 2014;14(8):679–88.
29. Keogh SJ, Long DA, Horn DV. Practice guidelines for sedation and analgesia management of critically ill children: a pilot study evaluating guideline impact and feasibility in the PICU. BMJ Open 2015;5(3):e006428.
30. Herring BO, Ader S, Maldonado A, et al. Impact of intravenous acetaminophen on reducing opioid use after hysterectomy. Pharmacotherapy 2014;34(Suppl 1):27S–33S.
31. Sinatra RS, Viscusi ER, Ding L, et al. Meta-analysis of the efficacy of the fentanyl iontophoretic transdermal system versus intravenous patient-controlled analgesia in postoperative pain management. Expert Opin Pharmacother 2015; 16(11):1607–13.
32. Lindley EM, Milligan K, Farmer R, et al. Patient-controlled transdermal fentanyl versus intravenous morphine pump after Spine surgery. Orthopedics 2015; 38(9):e819–24.
33. Ren ZY, Xu XQ, Bao YP, et al. The impact of genetic variation on sensitivity to opioid analgesics in patients with postoperative pain: a systematic review and meta-analysis. Pain Physician 2015;18(2):131–52.
34. Sehgal N, Smith HS, Manchikanti L. Peripherally acting opioids and clinical implications for pain control [review]. Pain Physician 2011;14(3):249–58.
35. Fleischman RJ, Frazer DG, Daya M, et al. Effectiveness and safety of fentanyl compared with morphine for out-of-hospital analgesia. Prehosp Emerg Care 2010;14(2):167–75.
36. De Gregori S, De Gregori M, Ranzani GN, et al. Morphine metabolism, transport and brain disposition [review]. Metab Brain Dis 2012;27(1):1–5.
37. Todd RD, McDavid SM, Brindley RL, et al. Gabapentin inhibits catecholamine release from adrenal chromaffin cells. Anesthesiology 2012;116(5):1013–24.
38. Brown SM, Campbell SD, Crafford A, et al. P-glycoprotein is a major determinant of norbuprenorphine brain exposure and antinociception. J Pharmacol Exp Ther 2012;343(1):53–61.
39. Slosky LM, Thompson BJ, Sanchez-Covarrubias L, et al. Acetaminophen modulates P-glycoprotein functional expression at the blood-brain barrier by a constitutive androstane receptor-dependent mechanism. Mol Pharmacol 2013;84(5): 774–86.
40. Sanchez-Covarrubias L, Slosky LM, Thompson BJ, et al. P-glycoprotein modulates morphine uptake into the CNS: a role for the non-steroidal anti-inflammatory drug diclofenac. PLoS One 2014;9(2):e88516.
41. Thibault K, Calvino B, Rivals I, et al. Molecular mechanisms underlying the enhanced analgesic effect of oxycodone compared to morphine in chemotherapy-induced neuropathic pain. PLoS One 2014;9(3):e91297.
42. Brophy GM, Bell R, Claassen J, et al, Neurocritical Care Society Status Epilepticus Guideline Writing Committee. Guidelines for the evaluation and management of status epilepticus. Neurocrit Care 2012;17(1):3–23.

43. Devlin JW, Roberts RJ, Fong JJ, et al. Efficacy and safety of quetiapine in critically ill patients with delirium: a prospective, multicenter, randomized, double-blind, placebo-controlled pilot study. Crit Care Med 2010;38(2):419–27.
44. De Witte JL, Alegret C, Sessler DI, et al. Preoperative alprazolam reduces anxiety in ambulatory surgery patients: a comparison with oral midazolam. Anesth Analg 2002;95(6):1601–6.
45. Green SM, Roback MG, Kennedy RM, et al. Clinical practice guideline for emergency department ketamine dissociative sedation: 2011 update. Ann Emerg Med 2011;57(5):449–61.
46. Kress JP, Pohlman AS, O'Connor MF, et al. Daily interruption of sedative infusions in critically ill patients undergoing mechanical ventilation. N Engl J Med 2000;342(20):1471–7.
47. Kudo S, Ishizaki T. Pharmacokinetics of Haloperidol: an update. Clin Pharm 1999;73(6):435–56.
48. Miller RD. Miller's anesthesia. 7th edition. Philadelphia: Churchill Livingstone;2010.
49. Pandharipande PP, Pun BT, Herr DL, et al. Effect of sedation with dexmedetomidine vs lorazepam on acute brain dysfunction in mechanically ventilated patients. The MENDS Randomized Controlled Trial. JAMA 2007;298(22):2644–53.
50. Riker RR, Shehabi Y, Bokesch PM, et al. Dexmedetomidine vs midazolam for sedation of critically ill patients. A randomized trial. JAMA 2009;301(5):489–99.

Tolerance and Withdrawal Issues with Sedatives in the Intensive Care Unit

Gina Riggi, PharmD, BCPS, BCCCP[a,*],
Antonia Zapantis, MS, PharmD, BCPS[b], Simon Leung, MS, PharmD, BCPS[c]

KEYWORDS

- Sedation • Tolerance • Intensive care unit • Iatrogenic withdrawal

KEY POINTS

- Patients admitted to the intensive care unit likely receive medications for pain and sedation.
- Tolerance is a common complication of prolonged analgesia and sedation administration.
- Guidance to identify and treat iatrogenic withdrawal has not been established.
- Practitioners need to recognize risk factors for iatrogenic withdrawal as well as implement prevention and treatment strategies.

INTRODUCTION

Appropriate pain management in critically ill patients is vital, because uncontrolled pain may compromise patient hemodynamics, prolong mechanical ventilation, and extend intensive care unit (ICU) care. An additional concern of inappropriate pain management is oversedation, a well-known complication that can prolong ventilator use and ICU stay.[1] Although analgesic and sedative medications remain essential for pain control and compliance with mechanical ventilation, practitioners often do not recognize that prolonged use of these agents may lead to tolerance, dependence, and eventually iatrogenic withdrawal.

Decreasing clinical effect of a drug after prolonged exposure, or tolerance, is a common complication of prolonged analgesia and sedation administration, resulting in a greater amount of the substance to maintain same therapeutic effect originally

This article is an update of an article previously published in *Critical Care Nursing Clinics of North America*, Volume 17, Issue 3, September 2005.
Disclosure Statement: The authors have nothing to disclose.
[a] Department of Pharmacy, Jackson Memorial Hospital, 1611 Northwest 12th Avenue, Miami, FL 33136, USA; [b] Department of Pharmacy, Delray Medical Center, 5352 Linton Boulevard, Delray Beach, FL 33484, USA; [c] Department of Pharmacy, Memorial Regional Hospital, 3501 Johnson Street, Hollywood, FL 33021, USA
* Corresponding author.
E-mail address: gina.riggi@jhsmiami.org

Crit Care Nurs Clin N Am 28 (2016) 155–167
http://dx.doi.org/10.1016/j.cnc.2016.02.010 ccnursing.theclinics.com
0899-5885/16/$ – see front matter

produced.[2–4] Functional cross-tolerance is a decrease in central nervous system (CNS) sensitivity to a similar substance. For example, tolerance to alcohol can lead to a decrease in normal response to the effects of sedatives.[2] There are several factors that affect the development of physical dependence, including tolerance, dose escalation, and prolonged treatment.

Dependence has referred to physical manifestations of withdrawal resulting from the body's physiologic adaptation to long-term drug use.[2] Such withdrawal has been described after seemingly brief use, for example, greater than 48 hours, but is more common with abrupt discontinuation.[5] High-dose benzodiazepine (BZD) administration increases the risk of developing moderate-to-severe withdrawal reactions. The concurrent administration of cross-dependent drugs also increases the occurrence of withdrawal reactions.[6] Once a patient develops tolerance and dependence, weaning from said medication is necessary to prevent iatrogenic withdrawal syndrome (IWS).

This group of symptoms has a negative effect on patient outcomes, including recovery and hospitalization.[4] Withdrawal can occur with stopping or reversing sedation after prolonged use and/or elevated doses of that substance and can vary according to the agent.[3,7] The onset and course of withdrawal are time-limited and are related to the type of substance and dose being taken immediately before cessation or dose reduction. Delayed clearance of active metabolites or the parent compound in patients with underlying renal or hepatic dysfunction may also delay the onset of the withdrawal symptoms.[7] Withdrawal is typically associated with 1 week or more of high-dose therapy.

Risk factors for opioid and BZD withdrawal include frequency, dose, and duration of administration. There are 3 different categories in which signs and symptoms of opioid and BZD withdrawal can be classified: CNS stimulation, gastrointestinal disturbances, and sympathetic nervous system activation (**Table 1**).[8]

In addition to dose and duration of sedatives administered, altered metabolism of critically ill patients can have an impact on the potential for tolerance, dependence, and withdrawal. Several sedative medications are generally highly protein bound and primarily eliminated by the liver, making them susceptible to a variety of drug interactions. Drug elimination is generally impaired, because hypoperfusion of liver and renal tissues slows drug delivery to these organs and thus may reduce excretion. For example, patients with an increased volume of distribution, such as those with cirrhosis, may accumulate midazolam.[9] Most sedatives and analgesics used for

Table 1
Signs and symptoms associated with opioid and benzodiazepine withdrawal

Central Nervous System		Gastrointestinal Disturbances	Sympathetic Nervous System
Agitation	Sleep disturbances	Nausea	Hypertension
Anxiety	Tremors	Vomiting	Tachycardia
Irritability	Movement disorders		Tachypnea
Restlessness	Hallucinations		Sweating
Pupillary dilation	Seizures		Fever

Data from Devlin J, Mallow-Corbett S, Riker R. Adverse drug events associated with the use of analgesics, sedatives and antipsychotics in the intensive care unit. Crit Care Med 2010;38:S231–43.

long periods of time are prone to drug accumulation and prolonged drug effects. In addition, medications, such as fentanyl and midazolam, accumulate in obese patients due to an increase in adipose tissue. Metabolic disturbances along with organ dysfunction can diminish drug efficacy or increase risk of toxicity. These issues are further complicated in the neonatal population.[10] This population has delayed drug elimination compared with adults with a large pharmacokinetic interindividual variability.[11]

These patient-specific characteristics illustrate the importance of continuous clinical monitoring and titration to the goal effect.[1] Knowledge of sedative and analgesic pharmacology is essential to the delivery of appropriate pharmaceutical care to critically ill patients.

The potential for opioid, BZD, and propofol withdrawal should be considered after high doses or more than approximately 7 days of continuous therapy. Doses should be tapered systematically to prevent withdrawal symptoms. Tolerance may develop more rapidly with continuous versus intermittent administration. In addition, patients are at a higher risk of developing delirium when analgesia and sedative medications are abruptly stopped after approximately 7 days of continuous therapy.[1] In the past decade, little has been published on the pathophysiology and management of withdrawal due to routine medications used in the ICU setting. Following is a summary of the occurrence of tolerance and withdrawal in the most common sedative medications used in the ICU setting.

BENZODIAZEPINES

BZDs have several different therapeutic properties allowing them to act as anxiolytics, hypnotics, muscle relaxants, anticonvulsants, and amnestics. BZDs exert their actions by attaching to γ-aminobutyric acid receptor on cells in the CNS, causing a reduction in cellular excitability.[5] This inhibition promotes sedation.[2] Chronic BZD administration results in down-regulation of receptors, leading to decreased pharmacologic efficacy and less CNS inhibition, indicating tolerance has occurred.[7] To achieve the same effect more BZDs are needed. BZD dependence clinical indicators include anxiety, confusion, dread, extreme agitation, fear, panic attacks, and seizures.[2]

It is important to have accurate medication use history to identify patients who are at higher risk of developing withdrawal syndrome due to cross-tolerance. Doses to produce adequate sedation need to be higher than traditionally used in patients who regularly take BZDs or who drank large amounts of alcohol prior to admission.[12] Although in this population physical dependency and withdrawal are considered results of what has been administered in the ICU, they may also result from medications patients received prior to admission. This is why it is vital to consider outpatient medication and social history when initiating sedatives. Manufacturer-recommended dose titration is necessary to provide the desired level of sedation.[7] Conversely, high doses of BZDs are needed to overcome any tolerance developed to achieve sedation during acute BZD or alcohol withdrawal.[2,13]

In a systematic review regarding the risk factors associated with iatrogenic opioid and BZD withdrawal in critically ill pediatric patients, the risk factors were categorized into 3 different groups: patient-level, process-level, and system-level factors (**Table 2**). Severity of illness also plays a role in the risk of IWS, with illnesses involving brain injury and ischemia at the highest risk. Overall, the strongest risk factors associated with IWS are duration of therapy and cumulative dose.[4]

The Withdrawal Assessment Tool–Version 1 (WAT-1) can be used to assess the potential and monitor for withdrawal in pediatric patients.[14] Available evidence

Table 2
Risk factors associated with iatrogenic opioid and benzodiazepine withdrawal

Patient Factors	Process Factors	System Factors
• Age • Severity of illness • Duration of therapy • Dose	• Institution sedation protocol • Drug choice • Mode of administration • Weaning • Multidrug use	• Protocol compliance • Bed availability • Interprofessional communication • Hospital-based sedative medication policies

Data from Best K, Boullata J, Curley M. Risk factors associated with iatrogenic opioid and benzodiazepine withdrawal in critically ill pediatric patients: a systematic review and conceptual model. Pediatr Crit Care Med 2015;16:175–83.

identifies IWS as a WAT-1 score of greater than or equal to 3. One study revealed that up to 68% of pediatric patients receiving at least 5 days of sedation and analgesia experienced IWS as defined by the WAT-1 tool.[15,16] Although there is not a scale developed for adults, several studies reviewing sedation strategies have identified the incidence of IWS. In 1 chart review, adult burn patients with inhalation injury receiving mechanical ventilation with continuous BZD and opioid infusions were evaluated to determine the IWS incidence. Eleven patients (age 37 ± 3 years), of 324 patients reviewed with lorazepam or midazolam use for greater than 7 days, were identified to have mild to severe signs and symptoms of withdrawal. Symptoms included confusion, diaphoresis, muscle twitching, picking motion, and seizures. A majority of these symptoms were mild and did not influence wean rate. Of note, 2 patients did experience BZD withdrawal seizures.

Cammarano and colleagues[17] reviewed the incidence of withdrawal symptoms in adult mechanically ventilated ICU patients. Twenty-eight patients met inclusion criteria and, of those, 9 met criteria for a diagnosis of acute withdrawal syndrome. BZD withdrawal symptoms included dysphoria, tremor, headache, nausea, sweating, fatigue, anxiety, agitation, increased sensitivity to light and sound, paresthesias, strange sensations, muscle cramps, myoclonus, sleep disturbances, dizziness, delirium, and seizure. Patients were younger (34.9 years ± 4.6 years vs 50.9 years ± 4.0 years; $P = .017$) and more likely to have acute respiratory distress syndrome (ARDS) (7 [77.8%] vs 5 [26.3%]; $P = .017$). Patients experiencing withdrawal were more likely to receive greater than 1 day of concurrent propofol ($P = .013$) or neuromuscular blocker (NMB) therapy ($P = .004$). Sedative and narcotic titration is more difficult in patients receiving concomitant NMBs because of their suppression of usual clues to assess sedation or pain. Also, these patients receive higher doses of sedatives and analgesics in an attempt to avoid undetected awareness and pain. There was no difference in specific opioid or BZD administered. In addition, withdrawal patients had longer periods of mechanical ventilation (39.6 days ± 7.1 days vs 21.3 days ± 4.8 days; $P = .049$), BZD duration (38.2 days ± 7.5 days vs 19.6 days ± 4.0 days; $P = .049$), and propofol duration (18.6 days ± 5 days vs 6.6 days ± 1.9 days; $P = .049$). This could be because ARDS increases mechanical ventilation duration. The withdrawal group had significantly higher mean daily doses of narcotic (6.4 mg ± 2.1 mg vs 1.4 mg ± 0.2 mg) and BZDs (37.8 mg ± 11.8 mg vs 11.1 mg ± 3.2 mg). Because tolerance can occur within days and in this study BZD mean duration was longer than the time required to develop tolerance and increased dose requirements, tolerance was likely. Also, though it was not statistically significant, withdrawal patients were weaned 2 times faster than nonwithdrawal patients. Extended ICU care for greater than or equal to 7 days and larger sedative doses increased acute IWS risk during drug weaning.[17]

Riker and colleagues[18] performed a prospective double-blind, randomized controlled trial conducted in ICUs at 68 medical centers to determine if dexmedetomidine (DEX) improved outcomes in mechanically ventilated patients compared with midazolam. One of the safety measures was the incidence of withdrawal-related events. Overall, 4.9% of DEX-treated patients and 8.2% of midazolam-treated patients experienced at least 1 event related to withdrawal within 24 hours after the respective medication was discontinued ($P = .25$).[18]

BZD withdrawal may produce an abstinence syndrome, including increasing anxiety, fear, dread, confusion, and agitation, with abrupt withdrawal increasing the risk for refractory seizures.[2] A retrospective chart review of more than 27,000 patients evaluated the incidence of new-onset seizures in the medical or surgical ICU during an 11-year period. Fifty-five patients (58% female) ranging from 31 to 87 years old were identified with new-onset seizures. Of those, 18 patients had sudden drug withdrawal (17 narcotics and 1 midazolam). The midazolam withdrawal patient had received 12 days of therapy. All seizures occurred within 2 to 4 days after sudden withdrawal and were generalized tonic-clonic seizures.[19]

PROPOFOL

Structurally unrelated to BZDs, propofol is a phenol derivative that exhibits sedative-hypnotic activity.[20,21] Propofol is considered a first-line sedative agent to achieve light sedation in the ICU setting. Some propofol properties making it an ideal sedative agent include rapid onset of action, short duration of effect, easy titration, minimal side effects, and absence of active metabolites. The exact mechanism of action is uncertain. It is postulated, however, to be similar to the action of BZD.[22] The incidence of tolerance is unpredictable and the mechanisms are thought to be complex and multifactorial. Pharmacokinetic tolerance, which results from a change in the absorption, distribution, metabolism, or excretion of a drug that effectively reduces the concentration of the drug at its receptors, produces no more than a 3-fold decrease in drug response. Pharmacodynamic tolerance results from adaptive changes so that the response to a given concentration of drug is reduced. This typically involves changes in the availability of drug receptor or receptor responsiveness (up-regulation or down-regulation), with varying magnitude.

There are only a few reports of propofol tolerance in adult ICU patients.[23–25] A small study on mechanical ventilated patients (n = 11) demonstrated that 27% of patients who received propofol concurrently with alfenanil for more than 5 days developed tolerance, which was defined as an increased infusion rate with an accompanying increase in blood concentration at a constant Ramsay score of 3 (patient responds to commands only).[23] It is suggested that extrahepatic clearance, increased volume of distribution, and severity of illness might contribute to the development of tolerance. In addition, 2 other studies (n = 22 and n = 9) have suggested that the development of tolerance tended to occur after 7 days of continuous propofol infusion.[24,25] It is difficult to extrapolate information from these studies due to the lack of detailed description of the study methodology and the variability among study subjects and environments. Total body clearance of propofol (91–156 L/h) in short-term and long-term infusions for anesthesia exceed normal hepatic blood flow, suggesting the possibility of pulmonary clearance.[21] Furthermore, cross-tolerance has not been reported in humans with propofol, other sedative-hypnotic agents, and other analgesics.

This may be explained by propofol's unique structure and pharmacologic properties, suggesting a separate receptor-binding site to induce the sedative-hypnotic effect. If propofol tolerance is suspected, the infusion could be discontinued or the rate decreased and another sedative could be added to achieve the desired sedation levels.[20] The lipid profile should be monitored for infusions beyond 48 hours and/or rate escalations due to apparent tolerance, because this could lead to elevated triglyceride levels.[26]

Although not recommended for use in pediatric ICU patients due to its increased mortality rate, propofol continues to be used in pediatric anesthesia outside the ICU arena.[27] Conflicting clinical data have been reported on the development of increased tolerance after repeated exposures over time for deep sedation or general anesthesia in small children with malignancies requiring high-voltage outpatient radiation therapy.[28–32] Caution should be exercised, however, in interpretation due to flaws of study design, small sample size, and patient variability. Until larger and well-controlled studies are conducted to confirm the safety in pediatric patients, the use of this agent in an outpatient sedation setting should continue to be under extreme caution.

Although considered safe and well tolerated in adults when used in short-term sedation, long-term administration of propofol has been associated with withdrawal syndrome that occurs with dosage reduction or an abrupt discontinuation of continuous infusion in critical care settings. There have been several cases of adverse events associated with IWS after propofol infusion.[22,33–36] Cawley and colleagues[22] reported a case of a severely burned, mechanical ventilated, septic patient, who received propofol for sedation due to difficulty in maintaining adequate sedation from lorazepam and morphine, who experienced withdrawal from weaning off propofol. On 2 separate occasions (days 108 and 113 of hospital stay), 6 and 39 hours after weaning off propofol, the patient experienced sudden symptoms of agitation, tremor, tachycardia, tachypnea, and hyperpyrexia. Both incidents were resolved by reinitiating propofol infusion at 5 μg/kg/min.[22] In adults, 2 reports have been documented of seizure activity 5 or 6 days after discontinuation of propofol.[33–35] This phenomenon may be related to propofol's conflicting anticonvulsant and neuroexcitatory activities, which require further investigation.[31,37,38] The propofol dose used in 1 patient was higher than in other published cases.[33] One 18-month-old burn patient experienced generalized twitching on withdrawal after being sedated and mechanically ventilated for 14 days.[36]

One small prospective study assessed adult ICU patients for delirium risk and signs and symptoms of withdrawal after the weaning of sedation in patients who required long-term opioid and sedation therapy while on mechanical ventilation support postoperatively. Patients with a known history of opioid, cocaine, alcohol, or BZD abuse were excluded. Patients were randomized to midazolam-based or a propofol-based sufentanil sedation regimens. Once sedation therapy was no longer necessary, the doses of midazolam, propofol, and sufentanil were gradually tapered by 30% every 6 hours. Withdrawal symptoms occurred more frequently in the midazolam/sufentanil group than the propofol/sufentanil group (33% vs 28%).[39] In addition, the opioid requirements were also increased in the group of patients receiving midazolam compared with propofol ($P<.10$), suggesting development of opioid tolerance when paired with a BZD.[39]

Based on the scant published data regarding propofol withdrawal syndrome, factors that can contribute to increased risk include prolonged infusion of greater than 5 days, symptoms that mimic BZD withdrawal, and rapid onset of withdrawal symptoms on discontinuation of propofol. Furthermore, it is speculated that age, gender, doses, comorbidities, and duration of weaning do not seem to play a major role.

It is difficult to provide conclusive recommendations for prevention of propofol dependence and withdrawal syndrome given the limited published data. To avoid undesirable events from long-term propofol use, it is important to avoid abrupt discontinuation of the infusion.[20] If potential propofol withdrawal syndrome is suspected, the previous infusion rate should be restarted before withdrawal symptoms occur. The infusion rate may then be decreased by approximately 10% every 6 hours if tolerated by the patient.[22] If withdrawal symptoms reappear, increasing the dosage or duration may be warranted. Unfortunately, consensus is still lacking on appropriate propofol tapering strategy in long-term ICU sedation and further work is needed in this area.

DEXMEDETOMIDINE

DEX, an imidazole derivative, is a highly selective α_2-adrenergic receptor agonist with 8 times higher the affinity to the α_2-adrenergic receptor than clonidine, an oral, nonsedating partial α_2-adrenergic receptor agonist/antihypertensive.[40,41] DEX produces sedation, analgesia, and anxiolytic effects without causing respiratory depression. Current guidelines recommend non-BZD therapy to achieve light sedation. Additionally, DEX is an effective sedative option for patients as they are weaned from mechanical ventilation support.[42] Although the Food and Drug Administration approval for this agent is sedation for a 24-hour period, numerous studies have demonstrated that DEX is safe to use for longer periods of time. In addition, there is a significant amount of literature supporting DEX use in conjunction with lorazepam for the prevention of alcohol withdrawal syndrome.

The sedative-hypnotic effect of DEX is suggested to be mediated through postsynaptic α_2-adrenergic receptors in the CNS. G_i-proteins allow opening of potassium channels and efflux of potassium ions, causing hyperpolarization of CNS cells, leading to a reduction in firing of excitable cells in the CNS. The diversity of pharmacologic effects of DEX may also include stimulation of phospholipase A_2 activity, increased Na^+/H^+ exchange, and elevated polyphosphoinositide hydrolysis through α_2-adrenergic receptor activation.[43,44]

As discussed previously, Riker and colleagues[18] reported 4.9% of DEX-treated patients and 8.2% of midazolam-treated patients experienced at least 1 event related to withdrawal within 24 hours after the respective medication ($P = .25$).[18] A prospective, open-label study was conducted at 10 Japanese investigational sites to assess the safety and efficacy of DEX as a sedative for more than 24 hours. One of the secondary safety endpoints was the incidence of withdrawal-related adverse events. Withdrawal symptoms were observed in 12% (9/75) of patients. All of the adverse effects were considered mild except for 1 patient who experienced a headache.[45]

Tolerance to DEX in humans has not been reported. Similar to clonidine, however, it has been documented extensively in animal studies.[46–50] Although the precise mechanism for the development of tolerance has not been fully elucidated, it may involve desensitization through receptor loss or receptor-effector uncoupling.[51] Tolerance to the hypnotic effect develops in chronic administration, approximately 7 days in animal models, with the effects becoming more pronounced after 14 days.[48–50] This response subsides on drug elimination. In contrast, tolerance to the analgesic effect of DEX occurs less frequently in rats compared with clonidine after chronic administration or at increased infusion rates.[50,52]

Cross-tolerance between DEX and BZDs has not been reported. Animal studies suggest, however, that cross-tolerance is unlikely to occur[50]; further studies are needed to confirm these findings in humans. Animal models have demonstrated a functional linkage between the *mu* opioid and α_2-adrenergic receptors.[53,54] In morphine-tolerant rats, the development of cross-tolerance to the hypnotic effects of DEX appeared after 4 days whereas cross-tolerance to the analgesic properties of DEX required a longer period of time.[52] This may be explained by a comparatively larger receptor reserve for the analgesic response in the spinal cord than for those needed for the hypnotic response.[48–50] Although the potential for cross-tolerance exists, it is difficult to interpret and extrapolate these data to humans because there are numerous limitations and the results have not been confirmed in clinical studies.

In theory, abrupt discontinuation of chronic DEX infusion may trigger withdrawal symptoms similar to those reported for clonidine. There is a large amount of data, however, on the use of DEX for sedation in critically ill patients, and rebound withdrawal symptoms are not common. Currently, guidelines on how to taper DEX have not been established and further work is required to determine appropriate tapering strategy for DEX after chronic administration.[1]

TREATMENT STRATEGIES

In general, whenever possible, withdrawal symptoms should be prevented and, if they occur, treated promptly.[5] It is recommended to taper medications that were administered at high doses or continuously for approximately 7 days.[1] Although there are no specific recommendations on tapering these medications, there are several studies that have used tapering schedules successfully. In patients who have been receiving these agents for less than 3 to 5 days, weaning analgesia and sedation medications may be done rapidly. One strategy is to titrate these medications by 10% to 15% every 6 to 8 hours.

When large doses of sedatives have been administered over long periods of time, a tapering regimen over several days to minimize withdrawal symptoms should be used.[55] It is also important to consider medication-specific characteristics when determining a tapering schedule. For example, although midazolam concentrations decline relatively slowly after an infusion, slow reduction of the infusion rate is preferred to abrupt discontinuation. This approach permits careful reappraisal of the underlying condition to avoid a sudden return of agitation, requiring sedative reloading and a general setback to the patients' progress.[55]

Because analgesics are often administered concurrently with sedatives and can mimic one another, it may be difficult to distinguish between opioid and sedative withdrawal. Opioid and BZD duration and dosing should be assessed to determine if overlap with oral agents should be initiated.[5] Data suggest the use of enteral methadone to prevent iatrogenic withdrawal, specifically in the pediatric population. Switching from intravenous fentanyl to oral methadone should account for the difference of the potency (fentanyl:methadone = 100:1), the difference in the half-life (fentanyl:methadone = 1:75–100 hours), and the oral bioavailability of methadone (75% to 80%). Increasing the dose to compensate for decreased oral bioavailability of methadone is not needed to prevent withdrawal symptoms. Cross-tolerance of opioids is not 100%; therefore, switching from one opioid to another may result in a decrease in total dose required when calculated on a standard potency ratio. BZD therapy for opioid withdrawal should be limited to treatment of seizures and extreme irritability and not as a replacement for opioid therapy.

When transitioning from continuous infusion sedation to intermittent dosing, the route of administration selected should be patient specific. It may be beneficial to convert to longer-acting oral agents to facilitate transition from the ICU to a step-down unit. The switch from intravenous midazolam to long-acting oral sedatives, such as lorazepam,

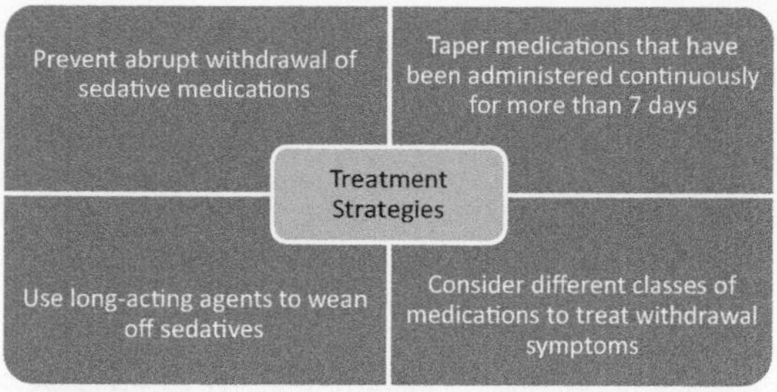

Fig. 1. IWS treatment strategies.

should account for the difference of the potency (midazolam:lorazepam = 1:2) and the difference in the half-life (midazolam:lorazepam = 1:6 hours).[56–74]

Clonidine may have a role in treatment of iatrogenic withdrawal. α_2-Adrenergic receptors mediate part of their pharmacologic actions through the activation of the same potassium channel as opioid receptors. Clonidine can be used as an adjunct for sedation and its role in the treatment of alcohol withdrawal symptoms. Based on withdrawal intensity, Korak-Leiter and colleagues[39] administered a clonidine infusion at 1 μg/kg/h to manage symptoms. **Fig. 1** reviews treatment strategies for IWS.

SUMMARY/DISCUSSION

Prolonged use of sedative medications continues to be a concern for critical care practitioners. Tolerance and withdrawal concerns increase the complexity of caring for critically ill patients. Dose requirements can be lessened and tolerance delayed with the use of pain or sedation scales, allowing for appropriate titration.[1]

Understanding of tolerance and withdrawal mechanisms begins with understanding of each sedative's pharmacology. Critically ill patients also have altered pharmacokinetic and pharmacodynamics profiles, making it difficult to predict response. Tolerance can occur with sedatives, even more rapidly with BZDs. Patient-specific factors, including outpatient medications, social history, alcohol abuse, prescription abuse, chronic exposure, increased drug clearance, and target receptor desensitization, all may contribute to the development of tolerance. In general, the best method for preventing IWS is to avoid abrupt discontinuation. It is imperative for all critical care nurses to collaborate with other practitioners to ensure that sedatives and analgesics are weaned properly to avoid withdrawal symptoms. When tapering these medications, it is important to consider the duration of use. Medications used for a short period of time may be titrated quickly; however, sedatives that were used for a prolonged period of time require a longer titration process to prevent withdrawal symptoms, possibly up to a few weeks. It is also important to take into account the combination of agents used for analgosedation; this combination may make it more difficult to predict a patient's response to titrating these medications. There are emerging data that there may also be a place for α_2-receptor agonists (clonidine and DEX) for the treatment of opioid and sedative withdrawal. Further research is still needed to better understand the development of tolerance and to determine the best approach in weaning therapy for commonly used sedatives. Society of Critical Care Medicine clinical practice guidelines do not make specific recommendations on the prophylaxis or treatment of opioid or sedative withdrawal. These guidelines recognize that patients who receive sedatives for a prolonged period of time should be weaned off these medications over several days to reduce the risk of drug withdrawal.[1]

REFERENCES

1. Barr J, Fraser G, Puntillo K, et al. Clinical practice guidelines for the management of pain, agitation, and delirium in adult patients in the intensive care unit. Crit Care Med 2013;41:263–306.
2. Puntillo K, Casella V, Reid M. Opioid and benzodiazepine tolerance and dependence: application of theory to critical care practice. Heart Lung 1997;26(4): 317–24.
3. Anand K, Willson D, Berger J, et al. Tolerance and withdrawal from prolonged opioid use in critically Ill children. Pediatrics 2010;125:e1208–25.
4. Best K, Boullata J, Curley M. Risk factors associated with iatrogenic opioid and benzodiazepine withdrawal in critically ill pediatric patients: a systematic review and conceptual model. Pediatr Crit Care Med 2015;16:175–83.
5. Taylor D. Iatrogenic drug dependence – a problem in intensive care? Intensive Crit Care Nurs 1999;15:95–100.
6. Fonsmark L, Rasmussen YH, Carl P. Occurrence of withdrawal in critically ill sedated children. Crit Care Med 1999;27(1):196–9.
7. Tobias JD. Subcutaneous administration of fentanyl and midazolam to prevent withdrawal after prolonged sedation in children. Crit Care Med 1999;27(10): 2262–5.
8. Devlin J, Mallow-Corbett S, Riker R. Adverse drug events associated with the use of analgesics, sedatives and antipsychotics in the intensive care unit. Crit Care Med 2010;38:S231–43.
9. Spina S, Ensom M. Clinical pharmacokinetic monitoring of midazolam in critically ill patients. Pharmacotherapy 2007;27:389–98.
10. Wagner BK, O'Hara DA. Pharmacokinetics and pharmacodynamics of sedatives and analgesics in the treatment of agitated critically ill patients. Clin Pharmacokinet 1997;33(6):426–53.
11. Jacqz-Aigrain E, Burtin P. Clinical pharmacokinetics of sedatives in neonates. Clin Pharmacokinet 1996;31(6):423–43.
12. Robb ND, Hargrave SA. Tolerance to intravenous midazolam as a result of oral benzodiazepine therapy: a potential problem for the provision of conscious sedation in dentistry. Anesth Pain Control Dent 1993;2(2):94–7.
13. Kunkel EJ, Rodgers C, DeMaria PA, et al. Use of high dose benzodiazepines in alcohol and sedative withdrawal delirium. Gen Hosp Psychiatry 1997;19:286–93.
14. Curley M, Harris S, Fraser K, et al. State behavioral scale: a sedation assessment instrument for infants and young children supported on mechanical ventilation. Pediatr Crit Care Med 2006;7(2):107–14.
15. Curley M, Wypij D, Watson S, et al. Protocolized sedation vs usual care in pediatric patients mechanically ventilated for acute respiratory failure: a randomized clinical trial. JAMA 2015;313(4):379–89.
16. Brown C, Albrecht R, Pettit H, et al. Opioid and benzodiazepine withdrawal syndrome in adult burn patients. Am Surg 2000;66(4):367–71.
17. Cammarano WB, Pittet JF, Weitz S, et al. Acute withdrawal syndrome related to the administration of analgesic and sedative medications in adult intensive care unit patients. Crit Care Med 1998;26(4):674–84.
18. Riker R, Shehabi Y, Bokesch P, et al. Dexmedetomidine vs midazolam for sedation of critically ill patients: a randomized trial. JAMA 2009;301(5):489–99.
19. Wijdicks E, Sharborough F. New-onset seizures in critically ill patients. Neurology 1993;43:1042–3.

20. Mirenda J, Broyles G. Propofol as used for sedation in the ICU. Chest 1995; 108(2):539–48.
21. Fulton B, Sorkin EM. Propofol. An overview of its pharmacology and a review of its clinical efficacy in intensive care sedation. Drugs 1995;50(4):636–57.
22. Cawley MJ, Guse TM, Laroia A, et al. Propofol withdrawal syndrome in an adult patient in thermal injury. Pharmacotherapy 2003;23(7):933–9.
23. Buckley PM. Propofol in patients needing long-term sedation in intensive care: an assessment of the development of tolerance. A pilot study. Intensive Care Med 1997;23(9):969–74.
24. Boyle WA, Shear JM, White PF, et al. Tolerance and hyperlipemia during long-term sedation with propofol. Anesthesiology 1990;73(3A):A245.
25. Foster SJ, Buckley PM. A retrospective review of two years' experience with propofol in one intensive care unit. J Drug Dev 1989;2(Suppl 2):73–4.
26. Jacobi J, Fraser GL, Coursin DB, et al. Clinical practice guidelines for the sustained use of sedatives and analgesics in the critically ill adult. Crit Care Med 2002;30(1):119–41.
27. Propofol [package insert]. Lake Forest, IL: Hospira; 2009.
28. Setlock M, Palmisano B. Tolerance does not develop to propofol used repeatedly for radiation therapy in children. Anesth Analg 1992;74:S278.
29. Setlock MA, Palmisano BW, Berens RJ, et al. Tolerance to propofol generally does not develop in pediatric patients undergoing radiation therapy. Anesthesiology 1996;85(1):207–9.
30. Deer TR, Rich GF. Propofol tolerance in a pediatric patient. Anesthesiology 1992; 77(4):828–9.
31. Keidan I, Perel A, Shabtai EL, et al. Children undergoing repeated exposures for radiation therapy do not develop tolerance to propofol: clinical and bispectral index data. Anesthesiology 2004;100(2):251–4.
32. Mayhew JF, Abouleish AE. Lack of tolerance to propofol. Anesthesiology 1996; 85(5):1209.
33. Valente JF, Anderson GL, Branson RD, et al. Disadvantages of prolonged propofol sedation in the critical care unit. Crit Care Med 1994;22(4):710–2.
34. Au J, Walker WS, Scott DHT. Withdrawal syndrome after propofol infusion. Anesthesia 1990;45(9):741–2.
35. Victory RA, Magee D. A case of convulsion after propofol anaesthesia. Anaesthesia 1988;43(10):904.
36. Imray JM, Hay A. Withdrawal syndrome after propofol. Anaesthesia 1991; 46(8):704.
37. Walder B, Tramer MR, Seeck M. Seizure-like phenomena and propofol. Neurology 2002;58(9):1327–32.
38. Marik PE, Varon J. The management of status epilepticus. Chest 2004;126(2): 582–91.
39. Korak-Leiter M, Likar R, Oher M, et al. Withdrawal following sufentanil/propofol and sufentanil/midazolam. Intensive Care Med 2005;31:380–7.
40. Bhana N, Goa KL, McClellan KJ. Dexmedetomidine. Drugs 2000;59(2):263–8.
41. Virtanen R, Savola JM, Saano V, et al. Characterization of the selectivity, specificity and potency of medetomidine as an alpha 2-adrenoceptor agonist. Eur J Pharmacol 1988;150(1–2):9–14.
42. Jones G, Murphy C, Gerlach A, et al. High dose dexmedetomidine for sedation in the intensive care unit: an evaluation of clinical efficacy and safety. Ann Pharmacother 2011;45:740–7.

43. Khan ZP, Ferguson CN, Jones RM. Alpha-2 and imidazoline receptor agonists. Anaesthesia 1999;54(2):146–65.
44. Ozaki M, Takeda J, Tanaka K, et al. Safety and efficacy of dexmedetomidine for long-term sedation in critically ill patients. J Anesth 2014;28:38–50.
45. Maze M, Scarfini C, Cavaliere F. New agents for sedation in the intensive care unit. Crit Care Clin 2001;17(4):881–97.
46. Paalzow G. Development of tolerance to the analgesic effect of clonidine in rats. Cross-tolerance to morphine. Naunyn Schmiedebergs Arch Pharmacol 1978; 304(1):1–4.
47. Yaksh TL, Reddy SV. Studies in the primate on the analgetic effects associated with intrathecal actions of opiates, alpha-adrenergic agonists and baclofen. Anesthesiology 1981;54(6):451–67.
48. Reid K, Hayashi Y, Guo TZ, et al. Chronic administration of an alpha 2 adrenergic agonist desensitizes rats to the anesthetic effects of dexmedetomidine. Pharmacol Biochem Behav 1994;47(1):171–5.
49. Reid K, Hayashi Y, Hsu J, et al. Chronic treatment with dexmedetomidine desensitizes α_2-adrenergic signal transduction. Pharmacol Biochem Behav 1997; 57(1–2):63–71.
50. Hayashi Y, Guo TZ, Maze M. Desensitization to the behavioral effects of alpha 2-adrenergic agonists in rats. Anesthesiology 1995;82(4):954–62.
51. Jones CR, Giembcyz M, Hamilton CA, et al. Desensitization of platelet alpha 2-adrenoceptors after short term infusions of adrenoceptor agonist in man. Clin Sci (Lond) 1986;70(2):147–53.
52. Bol CJJG, Danhof M, Stanski DR, et al. Pharmacokinetic-pharmacodynamic characterization of the cardiovascular, hypnotic, EEG and ventilatory responses to dexmedetomidine in the rat. J Pharmacol Exp Ther 1997;283(3):1051–8.
53. Hayashi Y, Guo TZ, Maze M. Hypnotic and analgesic effects of the α_2-adrenergic agonist dexmedetomidine in morphine-tolerant rats. Anesth Analg 1996;83(3): 606–10.
54. Kalso EA, Sullivan AF, McQuay HJ, et al. Cross-tolerance between *Mu* opioid and alpha-2 adrenergic receptors, but not between *Mu* and *Delta* opioid receptors in the spinal cord of the rat. J Pharmacol Exp Ther 1993;256(2):551–8.
55. Shafer A. Complications of sedation with midazolam in the intensive care unit and a comparison with other sedative regimens. Crit Care Med 1998;26(5):947–56.
56. Awissi D, Lebrun G, Fagan M, et al. Alcohol, nicotine and iatrogenic withdrawals in the ICU. Crit Care Med 2013;41:S57–68.
57. Jakob S, Ruokonen E, Grounds RM, et al. Dexmedetomidine vs midazolam or propofol for sedation during prolonged mechanical ventilation. JAMA 2012; 307(11):1151–60.
58. Tobias JD. Tolerance, withdrawal, and physical dependency after long-term sedation and analgesia of children in the pediatric intensive care unit. Crit Care Med 2000;28(6):2122–32.
59. Finkel JC, Elrefai A. The use of dexmedetomidine to facilitate opioid and benzodiazepine detoxification in an infant. Anesth Analg 2004;98(6):1658–9.
60. Maccioli GA. Dexmedetomidine to facilitate drug withdrawal. Anesthesiology 2003;98(2):575–7.
61. Multz AS. Prolonged dexmedetomidine infusion as an adjunct in treating sedation-induced withdrawal. Anesth Analg 2003;96(4):1054–5.
62. Angst MS, Koppert W, Pahl I, et al. Short-term infusion of the mu-opioid agonist remifentanil in humans causes hyperalgesia during withdrawal. Pain 2003; 106(1–2):49–57.

63. Compton P, Charuvastra VC, Ling W. Pain intolerance in opioid-maintained former opiate addicts: effect of long-acting maintenance agent. Drug Alcohol Depend 2001;63(2):139–46.
64. Tilson HA, Rech RH, Stolman S. Hyperalgesia during withdrawal as a means of measuring the degree of dependence in morphine dependent rats. Psychopharmacologia 1973;28(3):287–300.
65. VonVoigtlander PF, Lewis RA. A withdrawal hyperalgesia test for physical dependence: evaluation of mu and mixed-partial opioid agonists. J Pharmacol Methods 1983;10(4):277–82.
66. Davies MF, Haimor F, Lighthall G, et al. Dexmedetomidine fails to cause hyperalgesia after cessation of chronic administration. Anesth Analg 2003;96(1):195–200.
67. Kroboth PD, Smith RB, Erb RJ. Tolerance to alprazolam after intravenous bolus and continuous infusion: psychomotor & EEG effects. Clin Pharmacol Ther 1988;43:270–7.
68. Sury MRJ, Billingham I, Russell GN, et al. Acute benzodiazepine withdrawal syndrome after midazolam infusions in children. Crit Care Med 1989;17(3):301–2.
69. Carnevale FA, Ducharme C. Adverse reactions to the withdrawal of opioids and benzodiazepines in paediatric intensive care. Intensive Crit Care Nurs 1997;13:181–8.
70. van Engelen BGM, Gimbrere JS, Booy LH. Benzodiazepine withdrawal reaction in tow children following discontinuation of sedation with midazolam. Ann Pharmacother 1993;27:579–81.
71. Rosen DA, Rosen KR. Midazolam for sedation in the paediatric intensive care unit. Intensive Care Med 1991;17(Suppl):S15–9.
72. Finley PR, Nolan PR. Precipitation of benzodiazepine withdrawal following sudden discontinuation of midazolam. DICP 1989;23:151–2.
73. Hantson P, Clemesssy J, Baud F. Withdrawal syndrome following midazolam infusion. Intensive Care Med 1995;21:190–1.
74. Precedex [package insert]. Lake Forest, IL: Hospira; 1999.

Sleep Disturbances and Critical Illness

Roberta Kaplow, PhD, APRN-CCNS, AOCNS, CCRN

KEYWORDS

• Sleep disturbances • Critical care • Intensive care unit • Sleep

KEY POINTS

- Sleep is an essential part of life. It is required for its healing, defensive, and energy preserving functions.
- Disruption in sleep is often associated with critical illness. Alterations in sleep patterns, including sleep deprivation, are widespread problems experienced by intensive care unit (ICU) patients.
- The etiology of sleep deprivation in the ICU is multifactorial.

INTRODUCTION

Sleep is an essential part of life.[1,2] It is required for its healing, defensive, and energy preserving functions.[1] Despite its importance, sleep disturbances have been reported as a clinical entity for almost 4 decades. Several negative sequelae are associated with alterations in sleep patterns. Sleep disturbances are reported to continue following discharge from the intensive care unit (ICU) and the hospital, compromising patients' quality of life.[3] Several factors, including the ICU environment, have been implicated in the development of sleep disturbances. Multidisciplinary strategies to help mitigate sleep disturbances and optimize patient outcomes are described in this article.

WHY SLEEP IS NEEDED

Sleep disturbance is defined as "the perceived or actual alterations in nighttime sleep (both quantity and quality) with subsequent daytime impairment."[1(pp205)] Disruption in sleep is often associated with the onset of critical illness.[1,4] Alterations in sleep patterns, including sleep deprivation, are widespread problems experienced by patients admitted to the ICU.[3,5–15] Inferior quality of sleep compared with the sleep they receive at home is also reported.[5]

As far back as the early 2000s, patients have been reporting that inadequate sleep was among the most stressful aspects of their ICU admission.[13,16,17] Sleep is an essential element for recovery from critical illness and survival. It is also important

Funding: No funding support.
Disclosure: The author has nothing to disclose.
Emory University Hospital, 2184 Briarwood Bluff NE, Atlanta, GA 30319, USA
E-mail address: roberta.kaplow@emoryhealthcare.org

Crit Care Nurs Clin N Am 28 (2016) 169–182
http://dx.doi.org/10.1016/j.cnc.2016.02.005
ccnursing.theclinics.com
0899-5885/16/$ – see front matter

for emotional well-being and adequate cognitive, immunologic, and muscle function and healing,[1,7,10] and it affords the energy that patients need to partake in their treatment.[11] Adequate restorative sleep is also associated with decreased morbidity and with restoring health.[11,12]

NORMAL SLEEP ARCHITECTURE

Normal sleep is divided into 2 discrete phases: non–rapid eye movement (NREM) and rapid eye movement (REM) sleep. The phases are defined based on their distinctive electroencephalograph (EEG) characteristics.[9] NREM sleep is composed of 4 discrete stages from light to deep sleep. N1 and N2 (formerly stages 1 and 2, respectively) are considered light sleep. These stages precede deep slow wave sleep (SWS). N2 is thought to be most important for physiologic repair and the most restorative stage of sleep. N3 and N4 (formerly stages 3 and 4, respectively) are considered deeper sleep. REM sleep accounts for approximately 20% of total sleep time.

During REM sleep, there is an increase in cerebral and physiologic activity.[9] REM sleep increases in amount of time and intensity throughout the night. REM sleep is primarily a parasympathetic state with bursts of sympathetic activity. During the bursts, there is a risk for increases in heart rate and blood pressure and there is the greatest amount of risk for cardiac and respiratory instability. Patients are also at risk for cerebral ischemia and arrhythmias.[11]

During deep sleep, tissue repair is most effective. Energy sources are restored in deep sleep. There is also decreased ocular movement and decreased muscle activity during this time.[15]

Four to 6 repeated 90-minute cycles or periods of NREM and REM sleep comprise normal sleep architecture.[1,9,13,18] The percentages of total sleep time and the characteristics of the phases of sleep are shown in **Table 1**.

The sleep-wake cycle is controlled by 2 disparate processes. The drive for sleep (becoming sleepy, the onset of sleep, and sleep promotion) is controlled by process S, which is regulated by adenosine. Promotion of sleep is also regulated by secretion of melatonin from the pineal gland.[9] Sleeplessness is regulated by process C from the suprachiasmatic nucleus. Pathways from the suprachiasmatic nucleus inhibit release of melatonin in response to introduction of bright light. Other neurotransmitters that foster sleeplessness include dopamine, norepinephrine, histamine, serotonin, acetylcholine, and orexin.[9]

Table 1
Stages of sleep and associated characteristics

Stage of Sleep	TST (%)	Characteristics
N1	~2–5	Light sleep, start of sleep from being awake, drowsiness
N2	~45–55	Slow wave or deep sleep; can be easily awakened by noise
N3	~15–20	Restorative sleep, slow wave, deepest and most restful sleep
N4	~20–25	SWS, deep sleep, increased cerebral and physiologic activity, decreased muscle activity
R (REM)	~20	Restful sleep; primarily a parasympathetic state with bursts of sympathetic nervous system activity that can increase heart rate and blood pressure

Abbreviation: TST, total sleep time.
Data from Refs.[9,10,13,19]

TYPES OF SLEEP DISTURBANCES

Patients in the ICU may obtain an adequate number of hours of sleep while being treated. However, the sleep architecture is altered.[1,11] Patients' sleep in the ICU is interrupted, resulting in sleep deprivation. Patients may experience a decrease in total sleep time caused by several ICU environmental factors. These factors are discussed later. In addition to a decrease in total sleep time, sleep is reported as fragmented, there is excessive light sleep and decreases in slow wave and REM sleep, abnormal or loss of circadian rhythms, and frequent arousals and awakenings.[9,19,20] Poor sleep efficiency and sleep latency (taking longer to fall asleep) also occur,[9] and result in disproportionate daytime sleepiness. Patients also report poor sleep quality.[5]

Patients in the ICU may receive sedation to help decrease work of breathing or otherwise tolerate the required therapeutic modalities. Although it may seem that patients are asleep while receiving sedation, the type of sleep experienced is clinically and physiologically different from the sleep achieved without the use of sedative agents. Although patients appear to be asleep, they are getting poor sleep quality.[15]

CAUSE OF SLEEP DISTURBANCES IN THE INTENSIVE CARE UNIT

The cause of sleep deprivation in the ICU is multifactorial. Patients are increasingly vulnerable for sleep deprivation because of several environmental factors in the ICU, treatment modalities, patient demographics (eg, age), and medical conditions. Environmental factors include noise and light. Treatment modalities include frequent monitoring, medications, and mechanical ventilation. Patient conditions include age, medical conditions, and psychological and cognitive problems.

Environmental Factors

Noise

Several sources of noise have been implicated in the development of sleep disturbances in the ICU setting. These sources include alarms from monitoring devices (eg, cardiac monitors), infusion pumps, ventilator alarms and normal function of the ventilator, telephones ringing, beepers sounding, overhead paging, television, and health care providers conversing within patients' range.[2,7,10,11,19,21] In one study, noise was one of the 2 factors reported by patients that caused disruptions in sleep.[22] Kamdar and colleagues[9] reported that noise in the ICU frequently exceeds the maximum noise level recommended by the Environmental Protection Agency. Specifically, 45-dB and 35-dB levels recommended for day and night, respectively, are often exceeded and reported at more than 80 dB. This level is thought to contribute to sleep disruptions in the ICU. Delaney and colleagues[10] report that the World Health Organization recommends that hospital noise should not exceed 30 to 35 dB to minimize risk of sleep disturbances. They further report that the noise levels often exceed 70 dB and equate that level of noise to that created by motor vehicle traffic. Most noise is reported to come from health care providers.

Light

Exposure to artificial light in the ICU environment 24 hours a day can result in alterations in sleep patterns.[1,2,6,9–11,19,21] Elliott and colleagues[22] report that light was the other of 2 factors (with noise) that caused sleep disruption in the ICU. Exposure to artificial light is reported to stifle secretion of melatonin, which controls circadian rhythms.[10]

Treatment Modalities

Frequent monitoring

Frequent interruptions in sleep can result during monitoring and other patient care activities that occur around the clock in the ICU.[6,10,23] The need to obtain laboratory specimens, radiologic procedures, and other diagnostic studies further contributes to sleep disturbances in the ICU.[1] Patient care activities identified to contribute to sleep disruption in the ICU include performing patient assessments, wound care, bathing, measuring intake and output, and obtaining vital signs. Kamdar and colleagues[9] suggest that patients' sleep may be disrupted as many as 40 to 60 times per night. Because a full sleep cycle occurs in approximately 90 minutes, having 40 to 60 interruptions in sleep for patient care activities, it is easy to appreciate why patients report sleep deprivation.

Patients being maintained on bed rest are also at risk for sleep disturbances, This is thought to be related to loss of circadian rhythms, disruption of the sleep-wake cycle, and sleeping during the day when not participating in activities.[19]

Medications

Administration of various medications in the ICU can result in alterations in sleep architecture.[11] For example, opioids and benzodiazepines result in interrupted REM sleep.[6,11] Other classes of medications that reportedly cause sleep disturbances are those used for cardiovascular conditions, asthma, infections, depression, and seizures.[1] Medications used to regulate blood pressure, increase urinary output or cardiac output, or augment oxygen delivery are associated with changes in the activation of cortisol. The mechanism of action involves several neurotransmitter pathways and receptors that can also cause alterations in sleep patterns (**Table 2**).

Mechanical ventilation

Data suggest that the mode of mechanical ventilation received by the patient can affect sleep architecture and circadian rhythms. Specifically, high and low levels of pressure support can lead to sleep disruption in some patient groups (eg, patients with heart failure). Mechanical ventilation and high levels of pressure support can lead to patient/ventilator dyssynchrony, increased ventilatory effort, alterations in gas exchange, and air trapping, which can affect sleep quality.[1–3,5,6,9,11,24,25] Pressure support ventilation is further suggested to lead to decreases in carbon dioxide levels, which can cause central apneas and sleep arousal.[9,11]

Patients using mechanical ventilation reportedly experience increased levels of daytime sleepiness.[9] Disruptions for repeated patient assessments while mechanically ventilated contribute to sleep disturbances. Other aspects of mechanical ventilation that can cause sleep disturbances are sounding alarms, suctioning, increased ventilatory effort, and alterations in gas exchange.[9] In addition, discomfort from the endotracheal tube may affect sleep architecture.[1,9,22,25]

Noninvasive ventilation

Patients who receive noninvasive ventilation for more than 24 hours as a treatment of respiratory failure are reported to have sleep disturbances. Noninvasive ventilation is implicated in disruption of circadian rhythms and decreased REM sleep.[11]

Patient Factors

Patient demographics

A significant percentage of patients admitted to the ICU are older than 65 years.[26] There is a decrease in REM and deep sleep with age.[1] Older patients also have

Table 2
Effect on sleep of medications administered in the ICU

Classification of Medication	Medication	Effects on Sleep
Sedatives	—	Absence of REM sleep when administered concomitantly with NMBAs
Benzodiazepines	Lorazepam (Ativan) Alprazolam (Xanax) Diazepam (Valium) Midazolam (Versed)	Interrupted REM sleep; increases N1 and N2; decreases N3 and N4 sleep; suppress SWS; elimination of NREM sleep when used repeatedly; increased TST, decreased N3
	Dexmedetomidine (Precedex)	Increased N3, decreased sleep latency, decreased REM sleep
	Propofol (Diprivan)	Suppressed SWS; decreased REM sleep; elimination of NREM sleep when used repeatedly; increased TST; decreased sleep latency, decreased arousals once asleep, decreased sleep quality
Analgesics		
Opioids	Morphine sulfate Sublimaze (fentanyl)	Suppress SWS; increased NREM N2 sleep; interrupted REM sleep, decreased TST, decreased N3, increased arousals once asleep
NSAIDs	—	Decreased sleep efficiency and increased number of arousals; decreased TST; sleeplessness
Antipsychotics	Haloperidol (Haldol)	Increased TST, increased N3, increased sleep efficiency, decreased sleep latency, decreased arousals once asleep
	Olanzapine (Zyprexa)	Increased TST, increased SWS, increased REM sleep, increased sleep efficiency, decreased sleep latency, decreased arousals once asleep
	Risperidone (Risperdal)	Sleeplessness, increased TST and SWS, decreased REM sleep
Cardiac Medications		
β-Blockers	Propranolol (Inderal)	Decreased REM sleep; sleeplessness; bad dreams, increased arousals once asleep
	Amiodarone (Cordarone)	Bad dreams
	Norepinephrine (Levophed)	Decreased REM sleep, decreased N3
	Epinephrine (Adrenalin)	Decreased REM sleep, decreased N3
	Dopamine (Intropin)	Decreased REM sleep; decreased SWS, sleeplessness; decreased N3
	Phenylephrine (Neo-Synephrine)	Decreased REM sleep, decreased N3
Antidepressants		
Selective serotonin reuptake inhibitors	—	Decreased REM sleep; decreased TST, decreased sleep efficiency, increased SWS
Tricyclic antidepressants	—	Decreased REM sleep, increased SWS
Anticonvulsants	Phenytoin (Dilantin)	Increased sleep fragmentation

(continued on next page)

Table 2 (continued)		
Classification of Medication	**Medication**	**Effects on Sleep**
Antiinfectives		
Quinolones	—	Sleeplessness
Medications for asthma	—	Sleeplessness
Corticosteroids	—	Decreased REM sleep, decreased SWS, sleeplessness; decreased N3, increased arousals once asleep

Abbreviations: NMBAs, neuromuscular blocking agents; NSAIDs, nonsteroidal antiinflammatory drugs.

Data from Refs.[1,3,9–11,19]

increased sleep latency, less total sleep time, decreased sleep efficiency, and they are more likely to awaken than their younger counterparts. Combining age-related physiologic changes with other factors described here can result in alterations in sleep patterns and sleep deprivation.[1]

Patient conditions

Sleep disturbances have been associated with the presence of symptoms from respiratory, cardiac, renal, endocrine, and neurologic conditions. Diagnoses that result in ICU admission are associated with physiologic, emotional, and functional alterations and associated symptoms. These symptoms can result in sleep deprivation.[11] For example, patients with pulmonary conditions may desaturate during REM sleep. Similarly, presence of dyspnea, cough, or wheezing in patients with chronic obstructive pulmonary disease (COPD) may cause a decrease in REM sleep and duration of sleep. Patients with COPD also have prolonged sleep latency, decreased total sleep time, and increased arousals from sleep caused by hypoxia and hypoventilation.[9] Patients with obstructive sleep apnea can have fragmentation of sleep.[9]

Patients with diabetes report neuropathic pain, and awakening during the night to urinate; both can result in decreased and fragmented sleep. Patients with renal disease may develop sleep apnea or restless legs syndrome. In addition, presence of renal disease–associated uremia, itching, pain, or nausea can result in fragmented sleep.[9]

Patients with neurodegenerative or neuromuscular conditions are also at risk for fragmented sleep patterns and altered circadian rhythms. Patients following a stroke are at risk for sleep disturbances either from focal brain damage or from condition-associated medications or pain.[1]

A variety of other multisystem complications can disrupt normal sleep. For example, sepsis causes alterations in secretion of melatonin, increase in NREM sleep, and decrease in REM sleep, which can all contribute to poor sleep quality.[3,9] Patients with stroke or heart failure have altered breathing patterns, which are associated with disruptions in sleep. Presence of an alkalosis (increased pH) is associated with decreased SWS and more arousals.[11]

Psychological problems and cognitive dysfunction can lead to disruption in sleep. Anxiety, depression, and personality disorders are associated with alterations in sleep patterns.[1] Anxiety and stress related to critical illness, the ICU environment, or inability to verbalize (eg, from presence of an endotracheal tube) can cause sleep deprivation. Logically, pain is associated with patient awakening. However, even when patients do not appear to be awake, pain can interfere with normal sleep architecture.[9,11] In addition, there is an association between the presence of delirium and sleep alterations.

EFFECTS OF SLEEP DEPRIVATION ON PHYSIOLOGIC PROCESSES

Negative sequelae associated with sleep disturbance related to ICU admission have been well documented for many years.[5] Several organ systems are affected by sleep disturbances, which can affect recovery, prolong ICU length of stay, and increase mortality.[1,5,10–12,21,27] Complications of sleep disturbances by body system are shown in **Table 3**.

Changes in Temperature Regulation

Sleep contributes to temperature regulation. Thermoregulation follows a circadian pattern, with core body temperature highest in the later part of the day and lower just before the onset of sleep. There is a decrease in temperature sensitivity during NREM sleep, whereas REM sleep is associated with loss in ability to shiver or sweat.[9] Body temperature is lowest in the later part of sleep and temperature begins to increase just before awakening.[11] Alterations in sleep result in disruption of this circadian pattern.

Table 3
Complications of sleep disturbances by body system

Body System	Complications
Cardiac	Heart disease, hypertension (from increased catecholamine levels), increased sympathetic tone, decreased parasympathetic tone, increased risk for AMI (from endothelial disruption)
Respiratory	Variability in respiratory rate, pneumonia, delayed weaning from mechanical ventilation, impaired lung mechanics, increased oxygen consumption, increased CO_2 production, decreased respiratory drive, decreased inspiratory muscle endurance
Endocrine	Diabetes, altered endocrine responses; increased cortisol levels, increased T3, T4, and TSH levels; increased growth hormone and prolactin levels (may lead to muscle wasting and impaired immunity); hormonal effects; hyperglycemia; insulin resistance; altered glucose metabolism
Neurologic	Alterations in thermoregulation, fatigue, irritability, disorientation, hallucinations
Gastrointestinal	Alterations in metabolism, altered nitrogen balance, altered carbohydrate metabolism, catabolism, decreased glucagon levels
Psychiatric/cognitive	ICU psychosis, delirium, increased stress, psychological aberrancies, cognitive impairment, mood instability, depression, anxiety, decreased memory, decreased ability to concentrate, perceptual distortions
Hematologic/immunologic	Increased risk of cancer, production of proinflammatory mediators, impaired immune function, decreased natural killer cells, decreased T-helper cells, decreased phagocytosis activity, decreased leukocyte function
Other	Obesity, decreased quality of life, increased intensity of pain, excessive daytime sleepiness, decreased energy, reproductive changes

Abbreviations: AMI, acute myocardial infarction; TSH, thyroid-stimulating hormone.
Data from Refs.[1,2,5,6,10–12,15,19–21,30]

Changes in Respiratory Function

Breathing changes during each stage of sleep. There is a decrease in minute volume, tidal volume, and respiratory rate as the body shifts to N1 from wakefulness. As patients progress through NREM sleep, arterial carbon dioxide levels increase by 3 to 7 mm Hg. During REM sleep, there is inconsistency in tidal volume and respiratory rate. While sleeping, patients lose some of their hypoxic and hypercarbia drives to breathe; this is more pronounced during REM sleep.[9]

Many of the data on respiratory complications of sleep deprivation are from non-ICU patients with COPD. In these patients, a significant decrease in forced expiratory volume in 1 second, forced vital capacity, and maximal inspiratory pressure are reported. A decrease in ventilatory reaction to increased carbon dioxide (CO_2) levels has also been reported. In addition, sleep fragmentation increases the risk of upper airway collapse, which can result in obstructive sleep apnea.[9,10]

Changes in Cardiovascular Function

Changes in blood flow and electrical activity occur when patients are asleep. These changes contribute to ischemia and dysrhythmias in patients with a history of cardiac disease. During NREM sleep, a decrease in blood pressure, heart rate, and systemic vascular resistance occur because of increases in parasympathetic tone and decreases in sympathetic tone. During REM sleep, there is an increase in heart rate and venous return when patients inhale and decreases in heart rate and venous return when patients exhale.[9]

Changes in Gastrointestinal Function

When patients are asleep, there is an associated decrease in esophageal motility, swallowing, and production of saliva. Also, gastric acid secretion increases early in the sleep cycle.[9]

Changes in Endocrine Function

Production of growth hormone normally increases during the early part of N3 and is secreted during SWS, which results in synthesis of DNA and protein, and stimulates cell division. Prolactin levels increase during the second half of sleep. Both growth hormone and prolactin are needed for cell differentiation and proliferation. These processes contribute to tissue healing and physical restoration. Growth hormone and prolactin levels increase with critical illness; however, the beneficial effects may be countered by sleeplessness in the ICU, which augments catabolism. This process may result in muscle wasting and impaired immunity.[9,11] Cortisol levels increase in the early morning, are highest in late morning, and decrease at night. The lowest cortisol level occurs at the onset of sleep.[9] Cortisol, the stress hormone, has several important functions, including glucose and cell metabolism. Thyroid-stimulating hormone (TSH) has a similar pattern to cortisol, with the lowest level at the onset of sleep and inhibited by N3 sleep; levels of both hormones increase with sleep deprivation.[9]

The development of delirium is not well understood[10] but is proposed to be related to changes in release of melatonin and changes in circadian rhythms.[6] The development of hallucinations and perceptual distortions associated with sleep deprivation in the ICU have also been implicated.[19]

SLEEP MEASUREMENT TOOLS

Several methods are described to measure sleep. These methods include polysomnography (PSG), actigraphy, bispectral index (BIS), nursing assessments, and patient self-report. These methods are discussed in more detail later.

Polysomnography

PSG is considered the gold standard of sleep measurement. It is used in sleep research and is the only tool that is reliable for measuring sleep, particularly when evaluating patients with sleep disturbances.[19] This technology entails simultaneous recordings of EEG, electromyogram (EMG), and electro-oculography (recording of eye movement). Electro-oculography helps decipher NREM and REM sleep.[1] Issues surrounding use of PSG in the ICU setting are 2-fold. The equipment is bulky and testing is expensive because it requires skilled technicians to perform the testing and a sleep expert to interpret the data.[9–11] In addition, altered EEG patterns are common in sepsis, shock, hepatic encephalopathy, and acute kidney injury, as well as with several medications administered in the ICU setting (eg, sedation),[9] which makes it difficult to distinguish between the patient's physiologic condition and sleep.[19] Although there is an option for computer interpretation of PSG data, which may reduce some of the associated costs with this method, the reliability of the interpretation is questionable and its use has not been validated in the ICU patient population.[19]

Actigraphy

An actigraph unit is a small automated device worn on the wrist or leg that documents motion/gross motor activity.[1,9] The actigraph measures sleep efficiency and sleep-wake periods. Total sleep time, wake time, and sleep fragmentation data are reported. No data on presence of sleep efficiency or REM sleep are provided.[19] Because actigraphy is less costly, minimally invasive, and data easily interpreted, it holds several advantages compared with PSG.[10] However, a few concerns with using actigraphy are discussed in the literature. , For example, although the actigraph may be effective in measuring circadian rhythms and sleep fragmentation, no information about sleep architecture can be discerned from the device. Validity of results has been questioned because of the device's inability to discern differences between patients being asleep or awake and not moving, thereby overestimating total sleep time.[9,11] The device cannot approximate depth of sleep,[9] and has decreased ability to identify wakefulness.[11] It cannot be used on patients recovering from neuromuscular blockade, spinal cord injuries, or those with neuromuscular conditions that restrict spontaneous movements.[19] In addition, the actigraph has undergone only partial testing in the ICU setting.

Bispectral Index

BIS uses EEG leads and a foam sensor. It integrates EEG data on a scale of 0 to 100. Higher numbers equate to higher levels of consciousness.[9] This technology is typically used to assess patients' levels of sedation in the ICU and of anesthesia in the operating room. Scores of 90 to 100 equate to being awake. A patient with a score of 70 to 80 is considered unconscious; 60 to 70 is considered deep sedation; and less than 60 is considered under anesthesia.[19] BIS may estimate depth of sleep but sleep architecture may not be measured accurately.[9,11] Use of BIS to evaluate sleep in general or in the ICU has limited data. The advantages include that there is no need for a sleep expert to interpret the data and the data are readily available at the patient's bedside.[19]

Nursing Assessments

Patient observation by nurses is not an ideal way to quantify sleep in ICU patients. With this method, only total sleep time can be evaluated, which nurses characteristically overestimate.[15] Because they are not discernible through direct observation, nurses cannot distinguish NREM from REM sleep.[1] Also, nurses have difficulty distinguishing sleep from sedation.[19] To augment direct observation, there are valid and reliable instruments available to evaluate sleep in the critically ill, some for use in patients with cognitive impairment, making them suitable for ICU.[9] One example, the Richards-Campbell Sleep Questionnaire (RCSQ) is a 5-item survey that nurses can rate for the patient. The items evaluate sleep depth, sleep latency, number of awakenings, difficulty returning to sleep once awakened, and sleep quality. Each item is rated using a 100-mm visual analog scale.[9]

Patient Self-report

Patient assessment of quality and quantity of sleep can be evaluated by using one of several scales. In addition to the RCSQ, there is the Pittsburgh Sleep Quality Index, and the Verran and Snyder-Halpern (VSH) Sleep Scale. Each of the tools can measure sleep quality, sleep disturbance, sleep time, and sleep latency. In addition, the VSH Sleep Scale measures sleep fragmentation, length, latency, and depth with a 15-item evaluation. The Pittsburgh Sleep Quality Index and VSH Sleep Scale have a higher number of questions for the patients to answer than the RCSQ.[19] With the RCSQ, patients are able to quantify the number of hours of sleep they experienced the previous night and the quality of their sleep (better than average to worse than average).[15] Another instrument that has been used to evaluate sleep in critical ill patients is the Epworth Sleepiness Scale, which measures degree of sleepiness.[14] More recently, Sepahvand and colleagues[14] developed a valid and reliable 23-item instrument that measures sleep disturbances using a multidimensional framework. Items on the questionnaire are in one of 5 dimensions: sleep onset and continuity disorder, disorder in daytime functioning, sleep disturbances related to environmental factors (eg, noise, light, odors, required care interventions), sleep disturbances related to presence of cardiac disease (eg, acute coronary syndrome), and respiratory disorders during sleep (eg, obstructive sleep apnea). The instrument has been validated in patients in the coronary care unit with acute coronary syndrome; however, further refinement of the instrument in other critical illness and ICU settings is required.

Patient self-report of sleep has some degree of validity because patients are able to compare quality of sleep before, during, and after critical illness. In addition, daily sleep diaries and visual analog scales can be useful for self-report of various aspects of sleep.[1] Although patient self-assessment of sleep provides an ideal evaluation of sleep quality, there are reported disparities between patient self-report on quantity of sleep and total sleep time measured by PSG.[19]

STRATEGIES TO MINIMIZE SLEEP DISTURBANCES

Given what is known about risk factors and negative sequelae of sleep disturbances experienced by patients in the ICU, several strategies to mitigate alterations in sleep architecture are suggested for implementation by health care providers. These strategies are summarized in **Table 4**.

Patient Care Activities

Clustering of patient care activities is recommended to minimize sleep disruptions, promote sleep, and improve circadian rhythms.[4,8,9,12,27] Nursing routines should be modified to decrease sleep fragmentation and interruptions.[23] Some investigators recommend reducing environmental stimuli during certain hours of the night (eg, 12 midnight until 5 AM).[10,11,21] Clustering of activities and performing only

Table 4
Strategies to mitigate sleep disturbances

Cause of Disturbance	Strategies
Mechanical ventilation	• Collaborate with providers and respiratory therapist to use less pressure support and smaller tidal volumes • Observe for patient/ventilator dyssynchrony • Monitor for discomfort associated with endotracheal tube
Noise	• Reduce avoidable noise generated by bedside conversations, phone, and television to optimize maintenance of circadian rhythms • Keep doors closed, if possible • Decrease alarm volumes • Curtail discussions near the patient's bedside • Dissuade noisy, unnecessary activities (eg, emptying trash, changing linens) • Place beepers on silent/vibrate mode • Consider use of ear plugs • Whisper when in vicinity of patient's room
Light	• Dim lights at night • Keep lights on brighter setting during the day • If patient's room has a window, open blinds/curtains/shade during day for natural light exposure • Consider use of eye masks • Turn off lamps
Interruptions	• Limit interruptions at night to essential activities (eg, avoid bathing, routine dressing changes, routine linen changes) if feasible • Cluster activities to minimize sleep disruption, if patient is stable • Reduce environmental stimuli during certain hours of the night • Control visitation while patient is sleeping
Medications	• Minimize use of benzodiazepines and opioids as sleep agents • Avoid drugs that negatively affect sleep. Collaborate with provider to prescribe medications that interfere less with sleep architecture (eg, zolpidem [Ambien] and zaleplon [Sonata], which have less effect on deep NREM and REM sleep) • Consider judicious use of sedation • Promote comfort with pain medications, as indicated • Administer pain medication at least 30 min before bedtime • Advocate around-the-clock dosing of pain medication • Remove lines, tubes, catheters, and devices from under patient • Consider use of melatonin
Complementary therapies	• Massage • Foot rubs • Relaxation techniques (eg, music) • Read to patient (or have family read to patient) • Acupuncture • Mobilization to decrease muscle weakness, which has been shown to affect sleep • Optimize patient comfort
Temperature regulation	Avoid keeping room too warm or too cool (both interfere with sleep)

Data from Refs.[1,4,8–12,21,23,25,27]

activities that are clinically indicated and evidence based versus based on habit or routine is also recommended.[1–12,23]

Lights should be kept dim during sleep hours so as not to trigger arousal through melatonin suppression and disruption of circadian rhythms.[9] In contrast, increasing light sources during daylight or nonsleep hours contributes to normal cycles of day and night, which promote sleep.

Medications should be used for short amounts of time and efficacy evaluated on a regular basis. Health care providers should remember that an increase in total sleep time may be increased with sleep medications, but the quality of sleep does not necessarily improve.[1]

Mechanical Ventilation

Data suggest that mechanical ventilation causes sleep disturbances.[9] It has been recommended that, during the weaning process, patients should be reconnected at night while avoiding excessive pressure support and smaller tidal volumes to avoid central apnea, patient/ventilator dyssynchrony, and fragmentation of sleep.[5,9,11,12,25] Evaluation for patient/ventilator dyssynchrony should include assessment for use of accessory muscles of ventilation, anxiety/agitation, diaphoresis, tachypnea, tachycardia, and paradoxic abdominal movement.[28]

Melatonin

Decreased circadian rhythms and decreased melatonin secretions have been reported in patients receiving mechanical ventilation.[11] Melatonin controls the sleep-wake cycle and augments circadian rhythm. Administration of melatonin may enhance sleep for patients in the ICU by regulating circadian rhythms; however, more research is required.[6,10]

Complementary Therapies

Several complementary therapies have been suggested to help promote sleep. These therapies include massage, foot rubs, relaxation techniques (eg, music), reading, acupuncture, mobilization, optimizing comfort, and other nonpharmacologic interventions.[8,9,11,23,29] Massage may activate the parasympathetic nervous system, which results in a decrease in heart rate, blood pressure, respiratory rate, and stress. Researchers suggest that as few as 3 minutes of massage may have a therapeutic effect.[11] Stress has a negative impact on sleep; therefore, encouraging participation in activities that decrease stress may be beneficial.

Staff Education

Nurses may lack knowledge on the importance of sleep.[9] Without adequate knowledge on the value of sleep, nurses cannot prioritize interventions to promote good sleep architecture.[16] In addition to the benefits of quality sleep, education should include the detriments of poor sleep patterns and ways to maximize quality sleep. For example, educating staff on the impact of ambient noise promotes adherence to recommendations that decrease sleep disruptions from excessive noise.[10] A multifaceted, multidisciplinary approach is required to ensure optimal outcomes.

SUMMARY

Critically ill patients in the ICU report inferior quality of sleep. Poor sleep is associated with apprehension and distress, which affect patients' quality of life. Altered sleep architecture, quantity, and quality increases the risk for delirium and other complications, length of stay in the ICU, and mortality.[20] Sleep disturbances can also significantly affect patients' recovery from critical illness.[30] A multitude of factors contribute to sleep disturbances in the ICU, many of which are difficult to avoid. The complex, multisystem problems with which patients present when admitted to the ICU become the primary focus for the providers, which makes it easy to overlook the importance of sleep and consequently fail to implement sleep-promoting interventions.[31] Multidimensional approaches are necessary for enhancing patients' sleep while they are in the ICU, which is essential to recovery from critical illness with fewer complications and optimal outcomes.

REFERENCES

1. Matthews EE. Sleep disturbances and fatigue in critically ill patients. AACN Adv Crit Care 2011;22(3):204–24.
2. Roussos M, Parthasarathy S, Ayas NT. Can we improve sleep quality by changing the way we ventilate patients? Lung 2010;188:1–3.
3. Wang J, Greenberg H. Sleep and the ICU. Open Crit Care Med J 2013; 6(Suppl 1: M6):80–7.
4. Kanuert MP, Haspel JA, Pisani MA. Sleep loss and circadian rhythm disruption in the intensive care unit. Clin Chest Med 2015;36(3):419–29.
5. Ayas NT, Malhotra A, Parthsarathy S. To sleep or not to sleep, that is the question. Crit Care Med 2013;41(7):1808–10.
6. Bellapart J, Boots R. Potential use of melatonin in sleep and delirium in the critically ill. Br J Anaesth 2012;108(4):572–80.
7. Persson WK, Elmerhorst EM, Croy I, et al. Improvement of intensive care unit sound environment and analyses of consequences on sleep: an experimental study. Sleep Med 2013;14(12):1334–40.
8. Hofhuis JG, Langevoort G, Rommes JH, et al. Sleep disturbances and sedation practices in the intensive care unit—a postal survey in the Netherlands. Intensive Crit Care Nurs 2012;28(3):141–9.
9. Kamdar BB, Needham DM, Collop NA. Sleep deprivation in critical illness: Its role in physical and psychological recovery. J Intensive Care Med 2012;27(2):97–111.
10. Delaney LJ, Van Haren F, Lopez V. Sleeping on a problem: the impact of sleep disturbance on intensive care patients – a clinical review. Ann Intensive Care 2015;5:3. Available at: http://www.ncbi.nlm.nih.gov/pmc/articles/PMC4385145. Accessed November 19, 2015.
11. Pulak LM, Jensen L. Sleep in the intensive unit. A review. J Intensive Care Med 2016;31:14–23. Available at: http://jic.sagepub.com/content/early/2014/06/03/0885066614538749.full.pdf. Accessed November 19, 2015.
12. Eliassen KM, Hopstock LA. Sleep promotion in the intensive care unit–A survey of nurses' interventions. Intensive Crit Care Nurs 2011;27:138–42.
13. Delaney LJ, Van Haren F, Currie M, et al. Sleep monitoring techniques within intensive care. Int J Nurs Clin Pract 2015;2:114.
14. Sepahvand E, Jalali R, Paveh K, et al. Development and validation of sleep disturbance questionnaire in patients with acute coronary syndrome. Int Sch Res Notices 2014;2014. Available at: http://www.hindawi.com/journals/isrn/2014/978580/. Accessed November 19, 2015.
15. Ritmala-Castren M, Lakanmaa R-L, Leino-Kilpi H. Evaluating adult patients' sleep: an integrative literature review in critical care. Scand J Caring Sci 2014;28: 435–48.
16. Nesbitt L, Goode D. Nurses perceptions of sleep in the intensive care unit environment: a literature review. Intensive Crit Care Nurs 2014;30:231–5.
17. Tranmer JM. The sleep experience of medical and surgical patients. Clin Nurs Res 2003;12(3):159–73.

18. Bijwadia JS, Ejaz MS. Sleep and critical care. Curr Opin Crit Care 2009; 15(1):25–9.
19. Drouot X, Quentin S. Sleep neurobiology and critical care illness. Crit Care Clin 2015;31:379–91.
20. Boyko Y, Ording H, Jennum P. Sleep disturbances in critically ill patients in ICU: how much do we know? Acta Anaesthesiol Scand 2012;56(8):950–8.
21. Li SY, Wang TJ, Vivienne Wu SF, et al. Efficacy of controlling night-time noise and activities to improve patients' sleep quality in a surgical intensive care unit. J Clin Nurs 2011;20(3–4):396–407.
22. Elliott R, Rai T, McKinley S. Factors affecting sleep in the critically ill: an observational study. J Crit Care 2014;29(5):859–63.
23. Stuck A, Clark MJ, Connelly CD. Preventing intensive care unit delirium. A patient-centered approach to reducing sleep disruption. Dimens Crit Care Nurs 2011;30(6):315–20.
24. Roche-Campo F, Thille AW, Drouot X, et al. Comparison of sleep quality with mechanical versus spontaneous ventilation during weaning of critically-ill tracheostomized patients. Crit Care Med 2013;41(7):1637–41.
25. Watson PL, Ceriana P, Fanfulla F. Delirium: is sleep important? Best Pract Res Clin Anaesthesiol 2012;26(3):355–66.
26. Bell L. The epidemiology of acute and critical illness in older adults. Crit Care Nurs Clin North Am 2014;26(1):1–6.
27. Anderson JH, Boesen HC, Skovgaard OK. Sleep in the intensive care unit measure by polysomnography. Minerva Anestesiol 2013;79(7):804–15.
28. Gilstrap D, MacIntyre N. Patient-ventilatory interactions. Am J Respir Crit Care Med 2013;188(9):1058–68.
29. Tracy MF, Chian L. Nonpharmacologic interventions to manage common symptoms in patients receiving mechanical ventilation. Crit Care Nurse 2011;31(3): 19–28.
30. Sterniczuk R, Rusak B, Rockwood K. Sleep disturbance in older ICU patients. Clin Interv Aging 2014;9:969–77.
31. Talwar A, Liman B, Greenberg H, et al. Sleep in the intensive care unit. Indian J Chest Dis Allied Sci 2008;50:151–62.

The Impact of Liver and Renal Dysfunction on the Pharmacokinetics and Pharmacodynamics of Sedative and Analgesic Drugs in Critically Ill Adult Patients

Dinesh Yogaratnam, PharmD, BCPS, BCCCP[a,*],
Kristen Ditch, PharmD, BCPS[b], Kristin Medeiros, PharmD, BCPS[c],
Melissa A. Miller, PharmD, BCPS[d], Brian S. Smith, PharmD[e]

KEYWORDS

• Pharmacokinetics • Pharmacodynamics • Critical care • Sedatives • Analgesics • Renal • Hepatic • Dysfunction

KEY POINTS

- Sedative and analgesic drug therapy is often necessary to treat critically ill adult patients.
- Critically ill patients are at high risk for experiencing adverse events from sedative and analgesic drug therapy.
- Renal and hepatic dysfunction, which can occur frequently in critically ill patients, may alter the pharmacokinetics (PK) and pharmacodynamics (PD) of commonly used sedatives and analgesics.
- By anticipating how absorption, bioavailability, distribution, metabolism, and elimination might influence drug disposition for a given pharmacologic agent, a more tailored drug regimen can be designed.
- Frequent monitoring is required to ensure optimal safety and efficacy of sedative and analgesic drugs in critically ill patients, especially in the presence of liver or kidney impairment.

This article is an update of an article previously published in *Critical Care Nursing Clinics of North America*, Volume 17, Issue 3, September 2005.
Authors have no conflicts of interest to disclose.
[a] Department of Pharmacy Practice, Massachusetts College of Pharmacy and Health Sciences University, 19 Foster Street, Worcester, MA 01608, USA; [b] Department of Pharmacy, Neuro-Trauma Burn Intensive Care Unit, UMass Memorial Medical Center, 55 Lake Avenue North, Worcester, MA 01655, USA; [c] Department of Pharmacy, UMass Memorial Medical Center, 55 Lake Avenue North, Worcester, MA 01655, USA; [d] Emergency Medicine, New York-Presbyterian Hospital, 525 East 68th Street, New York, NY 10065, USA; [e] Specialty Pharmacy Services, UMass Memorial Shields Pharmacy, 55 Lake Avenue North, Worcester, MA 01655, USA
* Corresponding author.
E-mail address: Dinesh.yogaratnam@mcphs.edu

Crit Care Nurs Clin N Am 28 (2016) 183–194
http://dx.doi.org/10.1016/j.cnc.2016.02.009
ccnursing.theclinics.com

INTRODUCTION

ICU patients are at heightened risk for experiencing pain, anxiety, or delirium. These syndromes typically occur either as a result of critical illness or as a consequence of ICU care (catheter insertion or adjustment, mechanical ventilation, repositioning, and so forth). Agitated patients are at increased risk of stress-related morbidity, are less likely to tolerate mechanical ventilation, and are more likely to inadvertently remove intravenous catheters or endotracheal tubes. Sedative and analgesic drugs are often used to alleviate and prevent patient discomfort, reduce the risk of self-harm, and improve clinical outcomes.[1–3]

The benefits of these drugs, however, are counterbalanced by their adverse effects. Opioid analgesics are associated with constipation and respiratory depression, whereas dexmedetomidine and propofol are associated with hypotension and bradycardia. Benzodiazepines have been implicated in the development of ICU delirium, and the presence of delirium has been independently associated with prolonged duration of mechanical ventilation, increased length of ICU stays, and greater risk of death.[4,5] To minimize the risk of these adverse events, pharmacologic agents must be carefully selected, monitored, and titrated.[6] The presence of organ dysfunction in critically ill patients can complicate this process.

Hepatic and renal dysfunction is commonly observed in critically ill patients. The incidence of hepatic dysfunction has been shown to range between 11% and 54% among certain critically ill patient populations, whereas the incidence of acute kidney injury (AKI) has been shown to range between 5.4% and 19.2%.[7–9] Kidney and liver injury may also coexist, either acutely or chronically, in a given patient. Among patients with cirrhosis, the incidence of AKI may be as high as 50% to 70%, whereas the incidence of chronic kidney disease (CKD) has been reported as high as 13% and 17%.[10,11] Both the liver and the kidneys play a significant role in the PK of sedative and analgesic drugs. These PK changes, in turn, can affect the dose-response relationship and may lead to toxic effects or adverse events.

The liver is the primary organ responsible for the metabolism of drugs. The kidneys are primarily responsible for the elimination of drugs and their metabolites. Changes in liver or kidney function can have a clinically significant impact on the PK of sedative and analgesic medications that are used in the critical care setting. A drug's PK parameters, such as absorption, distribution, metabolism, and elimination, can be substantially altered as a result of either acute or chronic liver or kidney damage. As a result of these changes, the potency and duration of action for a sedative or analgesic drug dose may be markedly affected.

Unfortunately, most of the available PK data for sedatives and analgesics involve healthy volunteers or noncritically ill patients. Despite this limitation, it is important for clinicians to have a sound understanding of PK and PD principles to design, implement, and evaluate sedative and analgesic drug regimens for critically ill patients. This article provides an evidence-based review on the impact of hepatic and renal dysfunction on the PK and PD of select sedative and analgesic drugs used in the ICU setting. By understanding how PK parameters are affected by liver and kidney dysfunction, it may be possible to reduce the risk of unintended adverse drug events for this vulnerable patient population.[12–14]

The PK parameters for some of the more commonly used sedative and analgesic drugs are shown in **Tables 1** and **2**.

BIOAVAILABILITY

Bioavailability is the percentage of an administered drug dose that enters the systemic circulation. Definitions of this and other common PK terms are listed in **Box 1**. The oral

Table 1
Pharmacokinetics of commonly used sedative drugs

Drug	Metabolic Substrate	Active Metabolite	Hepatic Extraction Ratio	Protein Binding (%)	Elimination Half-Life (h)	Volume of Distribution (L/kg)
Dexmedetomidine	Glucuronyltransferase	None	High	93	1.8–3	1.49
Diazepam	CYP 2C19	Desmethyldiazepam	Low	99	19–54	1.1
Lorazepam	Glucuronyltransferase	None	Low	85–93	12	1.3
Midazolam	CYP 3A4	α-Hydroxymidazolam	Intermediate	95	1.8–6.4	1–2.5
Propofol	Glucuronyltransferase	None	High	98	1.5–12.4	60

Table 2
Pharmacokinetics of commonly used opioid analgesic drugs

Drug	Metabolic Substrate	Active Metabolite	Hepatic Extraction Ratio	Protein Binding (%)	Elimination Half-Life (h)	Volume of Distribution (L/kg)
Fentanyl	CYP 3A4	None	High	84	3.65	3.2–4
Hydromorphone	Glucuronyltransferase	Hydromorphone-6-glucuronide	Intermediate	71	2.65	1.22
Methadone	CYP 3A4	None	Low	89	23	3.6
Morphine	Glucuronyltransferase	Morphine-3-glucuronide Morphine-6-glucuronide	High	36	1.5–4.5	1–4

Box 1
Terms and definitions

Absorption	The process by which a drug enters the systemic circulation
Bioavailability	The percentage of an administered drug dose that enters the systemic circulation
Clearance	The volume of blood that is cleared of drug per unit time
Distribution	The movement of drug between body compartments. Usually, it describes the movement of drug from the systemic circulation to other compartments (fat tissue, extravascular fluid, brain tissue, etc.).
Elimination	The removal of drug from the systemic circulation
Extraction ratio	The fraction of drug presented to an eliminating organ, such as the liver, that is removed after 1 pass
Half-life	The amount of time required to reduce the concentration of drug by 50%. This usually refers to the concentration of drug in the systemic circulation.
Metabolism	The removal of drug from the body via biotransformation processes (enzymatic cleavage, conjugation reactions, etc.)
Pharmacokinetics	The absorption, distribution, metabolism, and elimination of drug through the body (ie, the effect of the body on the drug)
Pharmacodynamics	The physiologic response elicited by a dose of drug (ie, the effect of the drug on the body)
Steady state	The drug-dosing equilibrium when the rate of drug entering the systemic circulation equals the rate of drug leaving the systemic circulation (ie, rate of absorption = rate of elimination)
Volume of distribution	The degree to which a drug distributes from the systemic circulation to other compartments. The larger the Vd, the more a drug distributes to extravascular compartments.

bioavailability of most drugs is generally less than 100%. Oral bioavailability can vary widely depending on both the molecular characteristics of the drug and the relative acidity, function, and integrity of the gastrointestinal tract. Drugs administered orally are absorbed through the lining of the small intestine and enter into the enterohepatic circulation. Before entering the systemic circulation, the drugs pass through the liver and are exposed to hepatic metabolism. This process is often referred to as the *first-pass effect*. Unlike orally administered drugs, drugs that are administered intravenously do not undergo first-pass metabolism before entering the systemic circulation. Thus, intravenously administered medications are always 100% bioavailable.

When the liver has a compromised ability to metabolize drugs, such as in cirrhosis, the first-pass effect can be significantly diminished. For orally administered drugs that undergo extensive first-pass metabolism, systemic bioavailability may be considerably greater in the presence of cirrhosis. In a study involving 7 patients with a history of alcoholic cirrhosis and hepatic encephalopathy, the oral bioavailability of a single dose of morphine was found more than twice as high as in healthy controls.[15] Similarly, the systemic bioavailability of orally administered midazolam has been shown e significantly larger in patients with cirrhosis compared with healthy controls.[16]

DISTRIBUTION AND PROTEIN BINDING

Volume of distribution (Vd) is a relative term that describes the degree to which a drug moves from the systemic circulation to other body compartments, such as fat tissue, extravascular fluid, or brain tissue. It is typically expressed in liters or liters per kilogram of bodyweight. A drug's Vd is directly proportional to its half-life. Thus, increases in Vd can result in a prolonged therapeutic effect for certain sedative and analgesic drugs.

Drugs that are hydrophilic (water soluble) or highly protein bound have small volumes of distribution. Drugs with small volumes of distribution tend to remain mostly within the systemic circulatory compartment. Conversely, drugs that are lipophilic (lipid soluble) or are not significantly protein bound have large volumes of distribution. These drugs readily move out of the systemic circulation and into other body compartments.

Alterations in protein binding can have a profound effect on a drug's Vd. Plasma proteins, such as albumin and α_1-acid glycoprotein, serve as the primary source of oncotic pressure within the vascular space. Both of these proteins are produced by the liver, and their levels may be decreased in the setting of liver disease. As a consequence of lower concentrations of circulating plasma proteins, intravascular oncotic pressure falls. This leads to fluid shifting out of the intravascular space, which may increase the Vd of hydrophilic drugs. Patients with severe chronic liver disease, like alcoholic cirrhosis, often display increases in Vd as a result of impaired production of plasma proteins. Furthermore, critically ill patients often have reduced albumin due to malnutrition or acute illness.[17]

The PK of sedative and analgesic drugs may also be affected by protein binding. Protein-bound drugs exist in a state of equilibrium between unbound and bound drug states. Only the unbound (free) form of the drug is available to bind to its receptor and exert pharmacologic activity. In certain patient populations, such as those with burn injuries, the concentrations of these plasma proteins can increase or decrease, which can alter the amount of free, or unbound, drug. Diazepam, for example, is highly protein bound to albumin. As albumin levels decrease post–burn injury, the diazepam free fraction increases.[18]

Midazolam, a highly protein-bound drug, has been shown to lead to prolonged sedation in critically ill patients with hypoalbuminemia.[19] Conversely, morphine exhibits weak protein binding. Its Vd and half-life do not seem affected by hepatic dysfunction.[20]

The accumulation of fluid during renal failure can also have an impact on the extent of drug distribution throughout the body. As fluid accumulates, water-soluble drugs are able to diffuse with excess fluid into the extravascular space. This results in a reduced concentration of drug within the intravascular space that is available for metabolism and elimination, which reduces drug clearance. In a related phenomenon, alterations in fluid status can alter the concentration of drug that is presented to the pharmacologic site of action, resulting in a diminished dose-response relationship. Although changes in fluid status are often difficult to predict in critically ill patients with renal dysfunction, clinicians should be aware that sudden fluid shifts, like what may occur after a hemodialysis session, may impart a significant change in the PK and PD of sedative and analgesic agents.

METABOLISM AND CLEARANCE

Liver dysfunction can affect the metabolism of drugs by a variety of mechanisms. Reductions in functional hepatic blood flow, decreases in protein binding, and damage to liver cells can reduce the metabolism and clearance of drugs from the plasma.

The predominant hepatic mechanisms involved in the metabolism of sedatives and analgesics include cytochrome P-450 enzyme reactions (phase I metabolism) and conjugation reactions (phase II metabolism). These processes result in the biotransformation of drugs into water-soluble metabolites that can be eliminated through the kidneys or bile. Metabolites can be inactive, possess some degree of pharmacologic activity, or be toxic. Most active metabolites are generally less potent than their parent compound, but they can result in enhanced or prolonged pharmacologic activity if their elimination is impaired. Descriptions of the predominant metabolites of common ICU sedatives and opioids are listed in **Tables 1** and **2**.

Clearance is a term used to describe the volume of fluid that is completely cleared of a substance per unit of time. The clearance of sedative and analgesic drugs from the serum is largely dependent on the extent to which the liver can metabolize these agents. Hepatic clearance is the product of the hepatic extraction ratio and hepatic blood flow. The hepatic extraction ratio is the fraction of drug that is removed from circulation after 1 pass through the liver. With respect to hepatic clearance, drugs with a high extraction ratio (>70%) are significantly affected by changes in hepatic blood flow and less affected by changes in hepatic function. Conversely, drugs with a low extraction ratio (<30%) are much more sensitive to changes in hepatic function and less sensitive to changes in hepatic blood flow.[7,13,21] For example, fentanyl is a synthetic opioid analgesic with a high extraction ratio. The PK of intravenous fentanyl has previously been shown unaffected in surgical patients with impaired hepatic function secondary to cirrhosis.[22] The investigators attributed this lack of effect to the relatively preserved hepatic blood flow observed in the patients.

Drug-metabolizing enzymes and transporters are also present in the kidneys.[23–26] Patients with renal failure have been noted to have decreased expression and activity of these metabolic enzymes and transporters, resulting in decreased renal and hepatic drug metabolism.[27] A recent study showed that midazolam plasma concentrations were increased in critically ill patients with acute kidney disease. The increased midazolam concentrations were attributed to inhibition of hepatic cytochromes caused by kidney disease.[28]

ELIMINATION

Drug elimination can be increased or decreased in critically ill patients. The kidneys play the predominant role in eliminating drugs and metabolites from the systemic circulation. Renal drug clearance can be affected by nonrenal organ dysfunction (eg, heart failure or liver dysfunction), disease process (eg, sepsis, burn injury, or trauma), or an underlying condition (eg, malnutrition or chronic illness). Additionally, renal replacement therapies (RRTs), such as intermittent hemodialysis or continuous RRT (CRRT), techniques used to manage renal failure in critically ill patients, can enhance drug clearance.

Reductions in the glomerular filtration rate (GFR) may significantly reduce the elimination of drugs and drug metabolites. The active metabolites of morphine (morphine-3-glucuronide and morphine-6-glucuronide) and midazolam (glucuronidated α-hydroxymidazolam) have been shown to accumulate in critically ill patients with renal failure.[29,30] To avoid toxicity when using these medications in this patient population, clinicians should consider using alternative agents or empirically reduce the dose. The glucuronide metabolite of lorazepam has also been shown to accumulate in patients with renal failure, but this is of no clinical significance because the metabolite is neither active nor toxic at high concentrations.[31]

Increased renal clearance of medications, or augmented renal clearance (ARC), has been described in certain critically ill populations, such as young adult trauma patients, severe sepsis (early-stage) patients, and burn patients. This phenomenon has been associated with superphysiologic rates of renal clearance of β-lactam antibiotics.[32–34] ARC has also been associated with subtherapeutic vancomycin serum concentrations during the early stage of severe sepsis in adult critically ill patients.[35,36] ARC has been defined as the enhanced renal elimination of circulating solute. It is thought that enhanced cardiac output during periods of acute stress and systemic inflammation increases perfusion through the kidneys, which leads to the increased clearance of drugs.[36–38] In an observational study of ICU patients, the prevalence of ARC was approximately 65% within the first 7 study days of ICU admission.[37] Although the clinical implications of ARC have primarily been described with antibiotics, its effects on other renally eliminated drugs remain a concern. For example, it may be possible that patients with ARC may require more frequent dosing of morphine to maintain pain control than patients without ARC. Before specific recommendations can be made, however, further study is required to determine the clinical significance of ARC on sedative and analgesic drug dosing.

RENAL REPLACEMENT THERAPY

RRT has the potential to remove sedative and analgesic drugs from the systemic circulation. In general, water-soluble drugs with low molecular weight and minimal protein binding are readily removed during RRT. By contrast, lipophilic drugs with large Vds are only minimally removed. Because the PK of drugs during RRT can be complex, diligent monitoring for signs of efficacy and toxicity are often required to ensure optimal patient outcomes. Gabapentin, an anticonvulsant drug that is readily excreted by the kidneys and has low protein binding, is recommended for management of neuropathic pain in critically ill patients.[6] In a case series, gabapentin was used to manage neuropathic pain in patients receiving intermittent hemodialysis. Despite achieving good pain control, patients experienced toxicity (dizziness and somnolence) despite the use of a conservative dosing strategy. Further dose reductions were required to alleviate the adverse effects.[39,40]

CRRT can also have a significant impact on the concentrations of medications that are renally eliminated. The mode of CRRT, the degree of renal and/or liver dysfunction, and changes in blood and ultrafiltration flow rates can have an impact on plasma drug concentrations.[41] In a PK study of midazolam and its metabolites in ICU patients receiving CRRT, midazolam was not effectively removed by CRRT. The 1-hydroxymidazolam glucuronide metabolite, however, was effectively removed by CRRT.[42] These results are likely explained by the extensive protein binding of midazolam and the high water solubility of the glucuronide metabolite. Because the parent drug is poorly removed by CRRT, prolonged sedation may be seen in patients with severe renal failure who are receiving midazolam infusions.

ASSESSING ORGAN FUNCTION TO ADJUST DRUG THERAPY

Assessing renal and hepatic function in critically ill patients is a challenging but important step in appropriately designing sedative and analgesic drug regimens. The rate of elimination of renally eliminated drugs is often directly proportional to the GFR. The GFR is frequently estimated by creatinine clearance (CrCl), which is typically estimated using calculations that include serum creatinine and other patient-specific variables, but CrCl can also be directly measured by collecting urine over a standard period of time.[43–47]

CrCl measured through 24-hour urine collection can be cumbersome and error prone in an ICU setting. Noting the burden of 24-hour urine collection, Pickering and colleagues[48] evaluated the clinical utility of a 4-hour CrCl. Although the investigators found an increased likelihood of diagnosing AKI, the utility of using 4-hour CrCl to adjust renally eliminated drugs remains untested.

Equations that use serum creatinine to estimate renal function include the Cockroft-Gault, Modification of Diet in Renal Disease, and the Chronic Kidney Disease Epidemiology Collaboration. Although the Chronic Kidney Disease Epidemiology Collaboration has been associated with increased precision and reliability compared with Modification of Diet in Renal Disease, it has yet to be validated in critically ill patients.[49] Many conditions and situations in critically ill patients, such as hepatic dysfunction, fluctuations of creatinine production, and positive fluid balance, can alter the accuracy of any of these methods and overestimate GFR.[50] Despite these considerations, Cockroft-Gault remains the most used equation to guide drug dosing.

Assessing hepatic function in critically ill patients, for the purposes of drug dosing, can also be challenging. Although CrCl is a generally well-accepted indicator of renal function, there is no hepatic correlate that accurately reflects liver function. To help clinicians objectively assess liver function, several scoring systems have been developed. These scoring systems take laboratory data (bilirubin, albumin, and prothrombin time), clinical features (ascites, encephalopathy, and nutrition status), patient history (alcohol abuse), and patient status (hospitalized or ambulatory) into account to assess objectively the degree of hepatic impairment. Examples of such scoring systems, include the Child score, Child-Pugh score, and the Model for End-Stage Liver Disease score.[7,51–53] Although these scoring systems are useful in assessing the severity of liver disease and predicting mortality, they have not been validated as drug dosing tools.

SUMMARY/DISCUSSION

The presence of renal or hepatic dysfunction in critically ill patients can significantly alter the PK and PD of sedatives and analgesic drug therapy. Drug disposition can also be influenced by the presence of comorbid conditions, drug interactions, and the use of RRT. The impact of these changes on patient outcomes is often difficult to predict. To ensure optimal dosing of sedatives and analgesics and to promote positive therapeutic outcomes, regular and repeated clinical assessments need to be performed.[6] By anticipating these changes and routinely assessing the response to therapy, health care providers can offer effective treatment regimens that minimize adverse events.

REFERENCES

1. Reade MC, Finfer S. Sedation and delirium in the intensive care unit. N Engl J Med 2014;370:444–54.
2. Roberts DJ, Haroon B, Hall RI. Sedation for critically ill or injured adults in the intensive care unit. A shifting paradigm. Drugs 2012;72(14):1881–916.
3. Patel SB, Kress JP. Sedation and analgesia in the mechanically ventilated patient. Am J Respir Crit Care Med 2012;185(5):486–97.
4. Zaal IJ, Devlin JW, Hazelbag M, et al. Benzodiazepine-associated delirium in critically ill adults. Intensive Care Med 2015;41:2130–7.
5. Ely EW, Shintani A, Truman B, et al. Delirium as a predictor of mortality in mechanically ventilated patients in the intensive care unit. JAMA 2004;291(14):1753–62.
6. Barr J, Fraser GL, Puntillo K, et al. Clinical practice guidelines for the management of pain, agitation, and delirium in adult patients in the intensive care unit. Crit Care Med 2013;41(1):263–306.
7. Lin S, Smith BS. Drug dosing considerations for the critically ill patient with liver disease. Crit Care Nurs Clin North Am 2010;22:335–40.

8. Rimes-Stigare C, Frumento P, Bottai M, et al. Evolution of chronic renal impairment and long-term mortality after de novo acute kidney injury in the critically ill; a Swedish multi-centre cohort study. Crit Care 2015;19:221.
9. Bouchard J, Acharya A, Cerda J, et al. A prospective international multicenter study of AKI in the intensive care unit. Clin J Am Soc Nephrol 2015;10(8):1324–31.
10. Nadim MK, Durand F, Kellum JA, et al. Management of the critically ill patient with cirrhosis: a multidisciplinary perspective. J Hepatol 2015. http://dx.doi.org/10.1016/j.jhep.2015.10.019.
11. Warner NS, Cuthbert JA, Bhore R, et al. Acute kidney injury and chronic kidney disease in hospitalized patients with cirrhosis. J Investig Med 2011;59(8):1244–51.
12. Yogaratnam D, Miller MA, Smith BS. The effects of liver and renal dysfunction on the pharmacokinetics of sedatives and analgesics in the critically ill patient. Crit Care Nurs Clin North Am 2005;17:245–50.
13. Smith BS, Yogaratnam D, Levasseur-Franklin KE, et al. Introduction to drug pharmacokinetics in the critically ill patient. Chest 2012;141:1327–36.
14. Boucher BA, Wood GC, Swanson JM. Pharmacokinetic changes in critical illness. Crit Care Clin 2006;22:255–71.
15. Hasselstrom J, Eriksson S, Persson A, et al. The metabolism and bioavailability of morphine in patients with severe liver cirrhosis. Br J Clin Pharmacol 1990;29:289–97.
16. Pentikainen PJ, Valisalmi L, Himberg JJ, et al. Pharmacokinetics of midazolam following intravenous and oral administration in patients with chronic liver disease and in healthy subjects. J Clin Pharmacol 1989;29:272–7.
17. Marik PE. The treatment of hypoalbuminemia in the critically ill patient. Heart Lung 1993;22:166–70.
18. Martyn J, Abernethy D, Greenblatt D. Plasma protein binding of drugs after severe burn injury. Clin Pharmacol Ther 1984;35(4):535–9.
19. Vree TB, Shimoda M, Driessen JJ, et al. Decreased plasma albumin concentration results in increased volume of distribution and decreased elimination of midazolam in intensive care patients. Clin Pharmacol Ther 1989;46:537–44.
20. Bosilkovska M, Walder B, Besson M, et al. Analgesics in patients with hepatic impairment. Drugs 2012;72:1645–69.
21. Verbeek RK. Pharmacokinetics and dosage adjustment in patients with hepatic dysfunction. Eur J Clin Pharmacol 2008;64:1147–61.
22. Haberer JP, Schoeffler P, Couderc E, et al. Fentanyl pharmacokinetics in anaesthetized patients with cirrhosis. Br J Anaesth 1982;54:1267–70.
23. Klotz U. Pathophysiological and disease-induced changes in drug distribution volume: pharmacokinetic implications. Clin Pharmacokinet 1976;1:204–18.
24. Vree TB, Hekster YA, Anderson PG. Contribution of the human kidney to the metabolic clearance of drugs. Ann Pharmacother 1992;26:1421–8.
25. Gibson TP. Renal disease and drug metabolism: an overview. Am J Kidney Dis 1986;8:7–17.
26. Anders MW. Metabolism of drugs by the kidney. Kidney Int 1980;18:636–47.
27. Lalande L, Charpiat B, Leboucher G, et al. Consequences of renal failure on non-renal clearance of drugs. Clin Pharmacokinet 2014;53:521–32.
28. Kirwan CJ, Macphee IA, Lee T, et al. Acute kidney injury reduces the hepatic metabolism of midazolam in critically ill patients. Intensive Care Med 2012;38(1):76–84.

29. Milne RW, Nation RL, Somogyi AA, et al. The influence of renal function on the clearance of morphine and its glucoronide metabolites in intensive-care patients. Br J Clin Pharmacol 1992;34:53–9.
30. Bauer TM, Ritz R, Haberthur C, et al. Prolonged sedation due to accumulation of conjugated metabolites of midazolam. Lancet 1995;346:145–7.
31. Morrison G, Chiang ST, Koepke HH, et al. Effect of renal impairment and hemodialysis on lorazepam kinetics. Clin Pharmacol Ther 1984;35:646–52.
32. Akers K, Niece K, Chung K, et al. Modified Augmented Renal Clearance score predicts rapid piperacillin and tazobactam clearance in critically ill surgery and trauma patients. J Trauma Acute Care Surg 2014;77(3 Suppl 2):S163–70.
33. Carlier M, Carrette S, Roberts J, et al. Meropenem and pipercillin/tazobactam prescribing in critically ill patients: does augmented renal clearance affect pharmacokinetic/pharmacodynamics target attainment when extended infusions are used? Crit Care 2013;17:R84.
34. Claus B, Hoste E, Colpaert K, et al. Augmente renal clearance is a common finding with worse clinical outcome in critically ill patients receiving antimicrobial therapy. J Crit Care 2013;28:695–700.
35. Baptista JP, Sousa E, Martins P, et al. Augmented renal clearance in septic patients and implications for vancomycin optimization. Int J Antimicrob Agents 2012;39:420–3.
36. Campassi M, Gonzalez M, Masevicius F, et al. Augmented renal clearance in critically ill patients: incidence associated factors and effects on vancomycin treatment. Rev Bras Ter Intensiva 2014;26(1):13–20.
37. Udy A, Baptista J, Lim N, et al. Augmented renal clearance in the ICU: results of a multicenter observational study of renal function in critically ill patients with Normal plasma creatinine concentrations. Crit Care Med 2014;42:520–7.
38. Udy A, Roberts J, Boots R, et al. Augmented renal clearance: implications for antibacterial dosing in the critically ill. Clin Pharmacokinet 2010;49(1):1–16.
39. Spaia S, Tersi M, Sidiropoulou M, et al. Management of neuropathic pain in dialysis patients: an effective approach with gabapentin. Dial Transplant 2009;38(9):368–73.
40. Neurontin (gabapentin) [package insert]. NYC, NY: Pfizer; 2015.
41. Jiang S, Zhu Z, Wu X, et al. Effectiveness of pharmacist dosing adjustment for critically ill patients receiving continuous renal replacement therapy: a comparative study. Ther Clin Risk Manag 2014;10:405–12.
42. Bolon M, Bastien O, Flamens C, et al. Midazolam disposition in patients undergoing continuous venovenous hemodialysis. J Clin Pharmacol 2001;41:959–62.
43. Levey AS, Bosch JP, Lewis JB, et al. A more accurate method to estimate glomerular filtration rate from serum creatinine: a new prediction equation. Modification of diet in renal disease study group. Ann Intern Med 1999;130:461–70.
44. Gaspari F, Ferrari S, Stucchi N, et al. Performance of different prediction equations for estimating renal function in kidney transplantation. Am J Transplant 2004;4:1826–35.
45. Cockcroft DW, Gault MH. Prediction of creatinine clearance from serum creatinine. Nephron 1976;16:31–41.
46. Molitoris BA. Measuring glomerular filtration rate in acute kidney injury: yes, but not yet. Crit Care 2012;16(5):158.
47. Molitoris BA. Measuring glomerular filtration rate in the intensive care unit: no substitutes please. Crit Care 2013;17(5):181.

48. Pickering JW, Frampton CM, Walker RJ, et al. Four hour creatinine clearance is better than plasma creatinine for monitoring renal function in critically ill patients. Crit Care 2012;16(3):R107.
49. Sunder S, Jayaraman R, Mahapatra HS, et al. Estimation of renal function in the intensive care unit: the covert concepts brought to light. J Intensive Care 2014; 2(1):31.
50. Bragadottir G, Redfors B, Ricksten SE. Assessing glomerular filtration rate (GFR) in critically ill patients with acute kidney injury-true GFR versus urinary creatinine clearance and estimating equations. Crit Care 2013;17(3):R108.
51. Child CG. The liver and portal hypertension. Philadelphia: WB Saunders; 1964.
52. Pugh RN, Murray-Lyon IM, Dawson JL, et al. Transection of the oesophagusfor bleeding oesophageal varices. Br J Surg 1973;60:646–9.
53. Kamath PS, Wiesner RH, Malinchoc M, et al. A model to predict survival in patients with end-stage liver disease. Hepatology 2001;33:464–70.

Sleep and Mechanical Ventilation in Critical Care

Patricia A. Blissitt, PhD, RN, CCRN, CNRN, SCRN, CCNS, CCM, ACNS-BC

KEYWORDS

• Sleep • Sleep deprivation • Mechanical ventilation • Critical care • Sedation

KEY POINTS

- High-quality sleep of sufficient duration is essential to recovery from critical care illness.
- Pulmonary physiology changes with sleep.
- Mechanical ventilation may support or oppose patient effort and impact sleep.
- The patient's mechanical ventilation needs are dynamic, depending on the patient's awake-sleep state and many other factors.
- Research to date is limited with conflicting results; however, the critical care nurse must use what is known to optimize sleep for the mechanically ventilated patient in critical care.

INTRODUCTION

Sleep disturbances have long been recognized in critically ill patients.[1–5] More than half of all intensive care unit patients may experience sleep deprivation, both quantitative and qualitative.[6,7] Sleep is restorative and facilitates healing. Inadequate sleep may result in impaired immune response; decreased resistance to infection; negative nitrogen balance; protein catabolism; disturbances in wound healing; and cardiac, pulmonary, neurologic, and psychological complications.[4,7–10] Interruption in sleep is multifactorial, including pain, disease state, environment, pharmacologic agents, and clinical assessment and interventions, and much has been written about their contributions to sleep disturbances in critical care. Of more recent consideration is the impact of mechanical ventilation on sleep and the potential for sleep disturbances in critical care. This discussion focuses on the relationship between sleep and mechanical ventilation.

THE PHYSIOLOGY OF SLEEP AND BREATHING

Integral to understanding the relationship between sleep and mechanical ventilation is knowledge regarding basic sleep physiology. Sleep is a dynamic process that

This article is an update of an article previously published in *Critical Care Nursing Clinics*, Volume 17, Issue 3, September 2005.
No conflicts of interest to disclose.
Harborview Medical Center, Clinical Education Box 359733, 325 Ninth Avenue, Seattle, WA 98104, USA
E-mail address: pbliss@u.washington.edu

Crit Care Nurs Clin N Am 28 (2016) 195–203
http://dx.doi.org/10.1016/j.cnc.2016.02.002 **ccnursing.theclinics.com**
0899-5885/16/$ – see front matter

consists of non–rapid eye movement (NREM) stages and rapid eye movement (REM). NREM consists of N1, N2, and N3. Stage N3 is also referred to as slow wave sleep (SWS). In normal sleep, N1, N2, N3, and REM occur between four to six times each night with the first cycle lasting approximately 70 to 100 minutes and each subsequent cycle lasting 90 to 120 minutes.[10] The first and second sleep cycles are predominated by N3 (SWS) followed by later sleep cycles in which N2 and REM constitute a greater proportion of the sleep cycle. With each sleep cycle, the amount of time in REM increases. SWS and REM stages are considered the most restorative stages.[11] A normal sleep cycle typically consists of N1, N2, N3 (SWS) back to N2, and then REM repeatedly throughout the night.[10]

Breathing is a function of behavioral, chemical, and mechanical input. Control of breathing varies greatly during wakefulness and sleep. During the awake state, breathing is under behavioral influence and cortical input, which can override chemical and mechanical input. During sleep, chemoreceptors and reflexive respiratory feedback systems control breathing. Ventilation is controlled by chemoreceptors in the carotid bodies (for hypoxia and hypercapnia) and in the medulla (for hypercapnia) and by receptors in the chest wall, the Hering-Breuer reflex.[11,12]

PHYSIOLOGIC CHANGES IN BREATHING ASSOCIATED WITH SLEEP

Ventilatory responsiveness to hypoxia and hypercapnia decrease during sleep in healthy adults. The hypoxic ventilatory response in REM is less than in NREM sleep. The hypercapnic ventilator response is approximately 50% less in NREM sleep compared with wakefulness.[13] Dynamic changes in the thresholds at which the patient breathes during sleep result in instability.[11,12] Breathing has been described as arrhythmic or periodic at the onset of sleep with rises in $Paco_2$ resulting in arousals characterized by hyperventilation and a decrease in $Paco_2$. During stage N3 (SWS), breathing stabilizes but may become irregular again during REM. Tidal volumes and respiratory rates may vary.[14] In addition to changes in hypoxic and hypercapnic ventilatory responses, the muscle tone of the upper airway and accessory muscle decrease first during NREM and even more so during REM.[14] From awake to REM, the Pao_2 usually decreases from 2 to 12 mm Hg, arterial oxygen saturation diminishes about 2%, and the $Paco_2$ rises approximately 2 to 8 mm Hg.[11,14]

THE IMPACT OF MECHANICAL VENTILATION ON SLEEP

Several alterations in sleep architecture have been associated with mechanical ventilation, including changes in the total sleep time, sleep fragmentation (frequent arousals and awakenings), reduction of SWS and REM with an increase in stages 1 and 2 NREM sleep,[11] and disruption of the circadian rhythm.[15] Mechanical ventilation may contribute to sleep disturbances by destabilizing the patient's breathing, dyssynchronization between the ventilatory efforts of the patient and the machine, and inducing changes in the patient's respiratory efforts.[11,12] Indirect negative effects on sleep in association with mechanical ventilation include discomfort related to endotracheal intubation, noise from the ventilator alarms, and the use of sedation and analgesia to promote rest during mechanical ventilation.[11,12]

At least three issues have been identified around mechanical ventilation and its negative impact on sleep: (1) the mode, (2) the settings for a particular mode, and (3) the dynamic needs of the mechanically ventilated patient during any 24-hour time period. First, a pressure support ventilation (PSV) mode in which the patient's own initiation of inspiration is assisted at a preset level of pressure but no actual rate per minute may result in hyperventilation, followed by hypocapnia and central apnea.[16] The central apnea causes sleep fragmentation with arousals and awakenings.[4] PSV may require different levels of pressure at sleep versus an awake state. A lower level during sleep, allowing the $Paco_2$ to increase slightly, may minimize the risk of central apnea.[17] Adding dead space during sleep has also been shown to raise the $Paco_2$ slightly and improve the quality of sleep.[4]

In addition, a change of mode, such as from PSV to assist-control ventilation (ACV), also known as continuous mandatory ventilation, may allow for better sleep and rest of the respiratory muscles. In ACV the patient can trigger the ventilator to initiate a breath but each breath is assisted by the ventilator to ensure a set tidal volume or pressure. If the patient fails to trigger a preset number of breaths, the ventilator delivers a preset minimum number of breaths, at the preset volume or pressure.[16] ACV or continuous mandatory ventilation during sleep may allow for an increase in stages 1 and 2 initially followed by increases in SWS later during the night, which is consistent with normal sleep.[17,18] A comparison of polysomnographic recording consisting of electroencephalogram (EEG), electro-oculogram, tidal volume, rib cage, and abdominal excursion tracings in ACV and PSV demonstrates the greater number of arousals and awakenings in PSV compared with ACV in **Fig. 1**.[4]

In response to the dynamic and complex ventilatory needs of the mechanically ventilated patient throughout wakefulness and the various stages of sleep, advanced modes, such as proportional assist ventilation (PAV), proportional assist ventilation

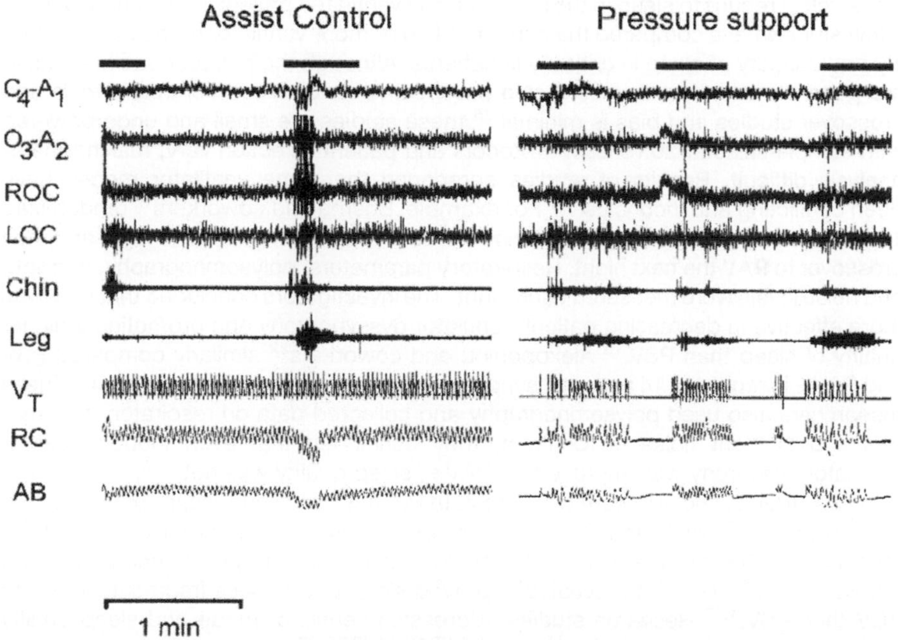

Fig. 1. Polysomnographic tracings during assist-control ventilation and pressure support in a representative patient. Electroencephalogram (*C_4-A_1, O_3-A_2*), electro-oculogram (*ROC, LOC*), electromyogram (*Chin* and *Leg*), integrated tidal volume (*V_T*), rib-cage (*RC*), and abdominal (*AB*) excursions on respiratory inductive plethysmography are shown. Arousals and awakenings, indicated by horizontal bars, were more numerous during pressure support than during assist-control ventilation. (*Reprinted* with permission of the American Thoracic Society. Copyright © 2016 American Thoracic Society. *From* Parthasarathy S, Tobin MJ. Effect of ventilator mode on sleep quality in critically ill patients. Am J Respir Crit Care Med 2002;166:1423–9. The American Journal of Respiratory and Critical Care Medicine is an official journal of the American Thoracic Society.)

plus (PAV+), and neurally adjusted ventilator assist (NAVA), have been developed. These modes in general detect the patient's efforts and then adjust the airway pressure accordingly to assist the patient with a more physiologic breath. In PAV the airway pressure is adjusted proportionally to the patient's efforts. As the patient's intrinsic inspiratory flow and tidal volume varies with each breath, so does the airway pressure of the ventilator.[19–22] PAV may improve patient-ventilator synchrony[19] and enhance sleep. However, it does not completely address the work of breathing. In contrast, PAV+ is an attempt to lessen the work of breathing by adjusting for the patient's lung compliance and elastance. Neurally adjusted ventilatory assist uses electromyographic input from a nasogastric catheter that measures diaphragmatic activity to provide feedback to the ventilator to assist in patient-ventilator synchrony by neuromechanical coupling. Neurally adjusted ventilator assist can operate effectively in the presence of auto-peep[16] and can eliminate ineffective breaths.[23,24] However, maintaining proper position of the nasogastric catheter is difficult and may add to the patient's discomfort and decreased quality of sleep. Repositioning of the catheter to provide adequate information about diaphragmatic movement to the ventilator may also result in repeated sleep disruption.

MECHANICAL VENTILATION AND SLEEP RESEARCH

Research in regard to sleep in the mechanically ventilated patient is rudimentary. Only a few studies have compared the impact of two or more ventilator modes on the quality and quantity of sleep in critically ill patients. Although the research methods used are generally sound, with most being prospective randomized controlled trials and crossover studies and bias is minimal,[25] these studies are small and underpowered with sample sizes of 20 or less. Protocols and patient selection vary, making meta-analysis difficult. Results of studies comparing the same ventilator modes have been conflicting and inconclusive. For example, Bosma and coworkers[19] randomized 13 patients in a medical-surgical intensive care unit to receive PSV one night and then crossover to PAV the next night. Respiratory parameters, polysomnography, and light and noise levels were measured each night. The investigators concluded that PAV was more effective in decreasing patient-ventilator dyssynchrony and promoting a higher quality of sleep than PSV.[19] Alexopoulou and coworkers[22] similarly compared PSV and PAV+ in regard to 14 patients' synchrony with ventilatory and sleep quality. These researchers also used polysomnography and collected data on respiratory parameters and ambient noise. In contrast, they concluded that even though patient-ventilator synchrony was improved on PAV+, sleep quality was not.

In two studies, findings were consistent. In Parthasarathy and Tobin[4] and Toublanc and coworkers,[17] ACV and PSV were compared with sample sizes of 11 and 20, respectively. Similar data were collected for each, including polysomnography and respiratory variables. Both revealed improved sleep quality (less fragmentation) with ACV than PSV.[4,17] Research studies addressing ventilator mode and sleep quality and quantity are summarized in **Table 1**.[4,17–19,21–23,25–28]

THE IMPACT OF SEDATION IN COMPLICATING SLEEP DURING MECHANICAL VENTILATION

A discussion on the effect of mechanical ventilation on sleep is lacking without some commentary about sedation. Sedation is likely used more often than not in the management of the critically ill mechanically ventilated patient, with the goals of patient-ventilator synchrony and enhanced comfort, rest, and sleep. The real impact of sedation on sleep is variable based on patient-specific factors but also perhaps

Table 1
Effects of mechanical ventilator mode on sleep

Author/Year	Study Design	Sample	Intervention	Control	Sedation	Findings
Bosma et al,[19] 2007	PRCT with crossover	13	PAV	PSV	Morphine, $\leq$0.01 mg/kg/h	PAV resulted in less patient-ventilator dyssynchrony and a better quality of sleep
Alexopoulou et al,[21] 2007	PRCT with crossover	17	PAV+	PSV	Approximately half were sedated	Patients not experiencing dyssynchrony during PSV, did not experience deterioration of sleep quality while on PAV+
Alexopoulou et al,[22] 2013	PRCT with crossover	14	PAV+	PSV	No	PAV+ improved patient synchrony but did not improve the quality of sleep
Parthasarathy & Tobin,[4] 2004	PRCT with crossover	11	ACV	PSV	Not stated	PSV results in hypocapnia, which results in central apnea and sleep fragmentation (decreased REM and absence of SWS)
Toublanc et al,[17] 2007	PRCT with crossover	20 (stable, nearing extubation)	ACV	PSV (low level)	No	Polysomnographic and perceived sleep quality was better on ACV than PSV (SWS present)
Cabello et al,[18] 2008	PRCT with crossover (three trials)	15	PSV (manual and automatic adjustment)	ACV	No	Sleep architecture abnormal, characterized by a brief REM and sleep fragmentation; ventilator mode did not affect the sleep pattern or the number of arousals or awakenings
Andréjak et al,[26] 2013	PRCT with crossover	13	Pressure controlled (CMV)	PSV (low)	No	PCV patients experienced improved sleep quality and quantity compared with low-level PSV
Roche-Campo et al,[27] 2013	PRCT with crossover	16	PSV	Spontaneous ventilation	No	In difficult to wean patients with tracheostomies, the quality of the patients' sleep was similar with or without mechanical ventilation; the sleep quantity was greater during mechanical ventilation
Delisle et al,[23] 2011	PRCT	14 (during weaning)	NAVA	PSV	No	NAVA increases REM sleep and decreases fragmentation and ineffective breathing efforts

Abbreviations: ACV, assist control ventilation; CMV, controlled mandatory ventilation; NAVA, neurally adjusted ventilatory assist; PAV, proportional assist ventilation; PAV+, proportional assist ventilation plus; PRCT, prospective randomized controlled trial; PSV, pressure support ventilation.

Data from Refs.[4,17–19,21–23,25–28]

related to dosing, administration schedule (continuous infusion versus intermittent, day versus night), duration, and pharmacokinetics. Interrupted sedation has been demonstrated to increase SWS and REM compared with continuous sedation.[29] In addition, the reported polysomnographic effects of various agents on sleep are variable from reference to reference, particularly in regard to propofol and dexmedetomidine as depicted in **Table 2**.[28,30–34]

ASSESSMENT OF SLEEP DURING MECHANICAL VENTILATION

In addition to the complexities described previously around attempts to understand and optimize sleep management of the critically ill patient on mechanical ventilation, the assessment of sleep during mechanical ventilation itself is controversial. The manual scoring of polysomnography, based on the American Academy of Sleep Medicine guidelines, includes EEG, electro-oculogram, electromyogram, chest, abdominal and extremity movements, airflow, pulse oximetry, and electrocardiogram data. These guidelines are the gold standard in sleep assessment.[35] However, Cooper and coworkers[36] and Ambrogio and coworkers[37] found that sleep by conventional polysomnographic scoring was severely disturbed in critically ill patients requiring ventilatory support. Up to 85% of polysomnographic findings in mechanically ventilated patients have been classified as atypical.[38] These findings have led clinicians and researchers to consider other means of assessment including automated (spectral analysis) EEG, the association between behavioral evidence of the sleep-wakefulness state and EEG, and the REM sleep alone,[37] in addition to the patient's perception of their sleep. Additional research around sleep assessment methods in the mechanically ventilated patient is needed, as is research directly related to management of mechanical ventilation.

CRITICAL CARE NURSING IMPLICATIONS

The implications for the critical care nurse and the entire interprofessional team including physicians, advanced practice nurses, respiratory therapists, and sleep medicine specialists around sleep in the mechanically ventilated critically ill patients are numerous. The critical care nurse must have a basic understanding of respiratory and sleep physiology and core knowledge of mechanical ventilation, including various ventilator modes and settings. That knowledge must extend to clinical expertise at the bedside in the nurse's assessment of the patient and actions related to the patient's

Table 2
Effects of sedation on sleep based on polysomnography

Medication	Effect on Sleep Based on Polysomnography
Opioids	Increased stage 2 NREM; decreased SWS, dose-dependent decreased REM, decrease in total sleep time; increased wakefulness after sleep onset
Benzodiazepines	Decreased SWS, decreased REM, decrease in sleep latency (time to onset of sleep), increase in total sleeping time; decreased wakefulness
Propofol (Diprivan)	Increased stage 2 NREM, decreased SWS, decreased *or* no effect on REM; decreased wakefulness, increased total sleep time; worsened sleep quality
Dexmedetomidine (Precedex)	Increased stage 2 NREM; increased *or* absence of SWS (when administered at night); decreased *or* total absence of REM when administered at night; shifting of sleep to nighttime if circadian rhythm disturbance; increased sleep efficiency

Data from Refs.[28,30–34]

response to respiratory and sleep interventions. Specific nursing care activities for sleep promotion are provided in the article by Kaplow elsewhere in this issue. The patient's ventilatory and sleep needs may change just as easily as their sleep-awake state during a 24-hour period and throughout their critical care stay.

Early recognition and management of deleterious signs of sleep deprivation in quality and quantity must be addressed immediately. The inability to provide high-quality sleep or sufficient duration may result in prolongation of mechanical ventilation, an increased length of stay, and potentially worse outcomes. An interprofessional team approach, including the nurse providing direct care to the patient, in the development of protocols, and clinical research will likely enhance the individual clinician's and entire team's expertise in regard to sleep, mechanical ventilation, and the critically ill patient.

SUMMARY

Strategies to fully optimize sleep in the mechanically ventilated patient are not fully known, which makes clinical decision-making all the more difficult. Factors affecting sleep are multifaceted, particularly in the critically ill patient requiring ventilatory support. Some modes and ventilator settings may be more beneficial in regard to sleep than others; however, the benefit of a given mode or ventilator setting may change throughout the day as the patient's awake-sleep state changes. Modes and settings that are changed manually or automatically in response to the patient's physiology with attention to individual variation will likely provide the patient the best opportunity for quality sleep of sufficient quantity.

REFERENCES

1. Hilton BA. Quantity and quality of patients' sleep and sleep-disturbing factors in a respiratory intensive care unit. J Adv Nurs 1976;1(6):453–68.
2. Aurell J, Elmqvist D. Sleep in the surgical intensive care unit: continuous polygraphic recording of sleep in nine patients receiving postoperative care. Br Med J 1985;290(6474):1029–32.
3. Richards KC, Bairnsfather LA. A description of night sleep patterns in the critical care unit. Heart Lung 1988;17(1):35–42.
4. Parthasarathy S, Tobin MJ. Sleep in the intensive care unit. Intensive Care Med 2004;30(2):197–206.
5. Bihari S, McEvoy RD, Matheson E, et al. Factors affecting sleep quality of patients in the intensive care unit. J Clin Sleep Med 2012;8(3):301–7.
6. Walder B, Haase U, Rundshagen I. Sleep disturbances in critically ill patients. Anaesthesist 2007;56(1):7–17.
7. Franck L, Tourtier J-P, Lobert N, et al. How did you sleep in the ICU? Crit Care 2011;15(2):408.
8. Friese RS. Sleep and recovery from critical illness and injury: a review of theory, current practice, and future directions. Crit Care Med 2008;36(3):697–705.
9. Bonnet MH. Acute sleep deprivation. In: Kryger MH, Roth T, Dement WC, editors. Principles and practice of sleep medicine. 5th edition. Philadelphia: Elsevier Saunders; 2011. p. 54–66.
10. Carskadon MA, Dement WB. Normal human sleep: an overview. In: Kryger MH, Roth T, Dement WC, editors. Principles and practice of sleep medicine. 5th edition. Philadelphia: Elsevier Saunders; 2011. p. 16–41.
11. Ozsancak A, D'Ambrosio C, Garpestad E, et al. Sleep and mechanical ventilation. Crit Care Clin 2008;24(3):517–31.

12. Psarologakis C, Kokkini S, Georgopoulos D. Sleep and mechanical ventilation in critically ill patients. In: Vincent JL, editor. Annual update in intensive care and emergency medicine. Cham (Switzerland): Springer International Publishing; 2014. p. 133–46.
13. Douglas NJ. Respiratory physiology: understanding the control of ventilation. In: Kryger MH, Roth T, Dement WC, editors. Principles and practice of sleep medicine. 5th edition. Philadelphia: Elsevier Saunders; 2011. p. 250–68.
14. Harrington J, Lee-Chiong T. Basic biology of sleep. Dent Clin North Am 2012;56: 319–30.
15. Gehlbach BK, Chapotot F, Leproult R, et al. Temporal disorganization of circadian rhythmicity and sleep-wake regulation in mechanically ventilated patient receiving continuous intravenous sedation. Sleep 2012;35(8):1105–14.
16. Hess DR, Kacmarek RM. Traditional modes of mechanical ventilation. In: Hess DR, Kacmarek RM, editors. Essentials of mechanical ventilation. 3rd edition. New York: McGraw-Hill; 2013. p. 50–9.
17. Toublanc B, Rose D, Glerant J-C, et al. Assist-control ventilation vs. low levels of pressure support ventilation and sleep quality in intubated ICU patients. Intensive Care Med 2007;33(7):1148–54.
18. Cabello B, Thille AW, Druouot X, et al. Sleep quality in mechanically ventilated patients; comparison of three ventilatory modes. Crit Care Med 2008;36(6):1749–55.
19. Bosma K, Ferreyra G, Ambrogio C, et al. Patient-ventilator interaction and sleep in mechanically ventilated patients: pressure support versus proportional assist ventilation. Crit Care Med 2007;35(4):1148–54.
20. Hess DR, Kacmarek RM. Advanced modes of mechanical ventilation. In: Hess DR, Kacmarek RM, editors. Essentials of mechanical ventilation. 3rd edition. New York: McGraw-Hill; 2013. p. 72–87.
21. Alexopoulou C, Kondili E, Vakouti E, et al. Sleep during proportional-assist ventilation with load-adjustable gain factors in critically ill patients. Intensive Care Med 2007;33(7):1139–47.
22. Alexopoulou C, Kondili E, Plataki M, et al. Patient-ventilator synchrony and sleep quality with proportional assist and pressure support ventilation. Intensive Care Med 2013;39(6):1040–7.
23. Delisle S, Ouellet P, Bellemare P, et al. Sleep quality in mechanically ventilated patients: comparison between NAVA and PSV modes. Ann Intensive Care 2011;1(1):42. Available at: http://www.annalsofintensivecare.com/content/1/1/42.
24. Verburgghe W, Jorens PG. Neurally adjusted ventilatory assist: a ventilation tool or a ventilation toy? Respir Care 2013;56(3):327–35.
25. Poongkunran C, John SG, Kannan AS, et al. A meta-analysis of sleep-promoting interventions during critical illness. Am J Med 2015;128(10):1126–37.
26. Andréjak C, Monconduit J, Rose D, et al. Does using pressure controlled ventilation to rest respiratory muscles improve sleep in ICU patients? Respir Med 2013; 107:534–41.
27. Roche-Campo F, Thille AW, Drouot X, et al. Comparison of sleep quality with mechanical versus spontaneous ventilation during weaning of critically ill tracheostomized patients. Crit Care Med 2013;41(7):1637–44.
28. Andersen JH, Boesen HC, Olsen KS. Sleep in the intensive care unit measured by polysomnography. Minerva Anestesiol 2013;79(7):804–15.
29. Oto J, Yamamoto K, Koike S, et al. Effect of daily sedative interruption on sleep stages of mechanically ventilated patients receiving midazolam infusion. Anaesth Intensive Care 2011;39(3):392–400.

30. Weinhouse GL, Watson PL. Sedation and sleep disturbances in the ICU. Anesthesiol Clin 2011;29(4):675–85.
31. Oto J, Yamamoto K, Koike S, et al. Sleep quality of mechanically ventilated patients sedated with dexmedetomidine. Intensive Care Med 2012;38(12):1982–9.
32. Kondilli E, Alexopoulou C, Xirouchaki N, et al. Effects of propofol on sleep quality in mechanically ventilated critically ill patients: a physiological study. Intensive Care Med 2012;38(10):1640–6.
33. Hanley PJ. Sleep in the ventilator-supported patient. In: Tobin MJ, editor. Principles and practice of mechanical ventilation. 3rd edition. New York: McGraw-Hill; 2013. p. 1293–305.
34. Alexopoulou C, Kondili E, Diamantaki E, et al. Effects of dexmedetomidine on sleep quality in critically ill patients. Anesthesiology 2014;121(4):801–7.
35. Berry RB, Brooks R, Gamaldo CE, et al. The AASM manual for the scoring of sleep and associated events. Version 2.2. Darien (IL): American Academy of Sleep Medicine; 2015.
36. Cooper AB, Thornley KS, Young GB, et al. Sleep in critically ill patients requiring mechanical ventilation. Chest 2000;117(3):809–18.
37. Ambrogio C, Koebnick J, Quan SF, et al. Assessment of sleep in ventilator-supported critically ill patients. Sleep 2008;31(11):1559–68.
38. Watson PL, Pandharipande P, Gelbach BK, et al. Atypical sleep in ventilated patients: empirical electroencephalography findings and the path toward revised ICU sleep scoring criteria. Crit Care Med 2013;41(8):1958–67.

Toward Solving the Sedation-Assessment Conundrum: Neurofunction Monitoring

DaiWai M. Olson, PhD, RN, CCRN, FNCS[a,*],
Kyloni Phillips, MSN, APRN, ACNP-BC, CNRN[a], Carmelo Graffagnino, MD, FNCS[b]

KEYWORDS

- Sedation assessment • Cerebral function monitoring • Neurofunction monitoring
- Neurocritical care nursing

KEY POINTS

- Sedation is required to facilitate a safe environment, medical care, nursing care, and to help blunt the patient from unpleasant experiences.
- Sedation interferes with the ability of nurses and physicians to obtain a comprehensive neurologic examination.
- In conflict with the purpose of sedation, intermittent observational (subjective) sedation assessment requires that the patient be stimulated to a point of arousal.
- Neurofunction monitors are an adjunct to sedation assessment by providing continuous data regarding the patient's state of arousal without requiring stimulation.
- A more balanced approach to sedation assessment may help alleviate the unwanted effects of stopping sedation in order to obtain a neurologic examination.

INTRODUCTION

The sedation-assessment conundrum[1] describes 2 vital but opposing forces that exist when assessing critically ill patients with neurologic illness or injury. The need for sedation is in opposition to the need for a sedation-free neurologic examination (neuroexamination). Sedation may be required to facilitate ventilatory and hemodynamic stability or to maintain a safe environment for the patient and staff.[2,3] However, sedation blunts the neurologic response. Therefore, the administration of sedatives must be interrupted in order to obtain a comprehensive neuroexamination.

This article is an update of an article previously published in *Critical Care Nursing Clinics*, Volume 17, Issue 3, September 2005.
Disclosure: The authors have nothing to disclose.
[a] Department of Neurology and Neurotherapeutics, University of Texas Southwestern, 5323 Harry Hines Boulevard, Dallas, TX 75390-8897, USA; [b] Department of Neurology, Duke University, 2100 Erwin Road, Durham, NC 27705, USA
* Corresponding author.
E-mail address: DaiWai.Olson@UTSouthwestern.edu

Crit Care Nurs Clin N Am 28 (2016) 205–216
http://dx.doi.org/10.1016/j.cnc.2016.02.007 ccnursing.theclinics.com
0899-5885/16/$ – see front matter

Determining the best practice for optimizing sedation continues to be a subject of debate.[4,5] Stopping sedation altogether, especially abruptly, may cause worsening of the injury and is controversial.[6] In the perfect setting, all patients would receive no more and no less sedation than is required to meet their needs at any moment. Traditional methods of sedation assessment rely largely on intermittent assessments designed to determine the minimum level of stimulus required to elicit a response.[7] Neurofunction monitors have been shown to provide additional information beyond what is obtained through a subjective neuroexamination.

DEFINING THE SEDATION-ASSESSMENT CONUNDRUM

Much of what clinicians (well-intentioned health care practitioners) do in the name of good medical assessment carries the risk of defeating good medical management. For example, consider a patient with a large left hemispheric stroke who is unable to protect her own airway. The patient is orally intubated and receives continuous intravenous (IV) sedation to facilitate mechanical ventilation. However, she is also subjected to serial neuroexaminations to trend her functional status. Knowing that sedation may blunt neurologic function, and because even a small change in her level of neurologic function could result in a profound need for medical intervention, the neuroexamination is performed without sedation.

Without sedation, the patient may be confused, combative, and have long periods of ventilator noncompliance. This situation places the patient at higher risk of injury from device self-removal, hypertension, and increased intracranial pressure (ICP). This situation also places the staff at risk of physical harm from a combative patient. However, with adequate sedation it is inappropriate to assume that any change in neurologic functioning is or is not related to a reversible neurologic condition (eg, seizure, cerebral edema, cerebral ischemia). Hence, the staff face a conundrum: how best can the risks of inadequate sedation be minimized without sacrificing the ability to obtain a comprehensive neuroexamination?

SEDATION

The reasons for sedation have remained fairly well defined for more than a decade: to prevent injury, facilitate care, and blunt psychological stress.[8] When sedation is indicated, practitioners must then determine a target for the depth of sedation. A key aspect of the guidelines for sedation management is the need to set, and regularly redefine, that target. In the intensive care unit (ICU) setting, there are a variety of reasons why clinicians might choose to chemically sedate a patient.

The first reason is that the patient, if left without adequate sedation, may cause injury to the patient or to others. This situation may include removal of medically necessary monitoring or support devices as well as causing injury to the staff members caring for them while they are in a state of agitation or delirium. Another major reason for sedating a patient is to facilitate the medical goals set for the patient; for example, maintaining hemodynamic stability, increasing ventilatory compliance, and controlling ICP.[9] Critically ill patients who have dangerous neurologic instability from minimal stimulation can have lasting harmful effects if exposed to extremely painful noxious stimuli for an extended period. Proper sedation is the only answer in preventing iatrogenic induction of a harmful metabolic crisis in response to the stimulus put upon a critically ill undersedated patient.

The third reason for sedating a patient is for humanitarian intentions. Adequate sedation of critically ill patients also becomes paramount when an individual is inflicted with a barrage of noxious stimuli and invasive procedures, such as the insertion of ICP monitoring devices or placement of medically necessary, but invasive, catheters. All patients treated with neuromuscular blocking agents should be concurrently treated with sedative medications to avoid the mental distress associated with total body paralysis.[10] Adequate sedation also results in a degree of induced amnesia for the events associated with the intensive care admission, thus protecting the patient against the long-term emotional stress of the acute illness.[11] Although each of these 3 reasons is valid enough to justify sedation, the needs often overlap.

The reason for sedation must be individualized to the needs of the patient and clearly communicated to all members of the ICU team.[12] If the indication for sedation is one of injury prevention, a lighter state of sedation is likely indicated, such that the patient is cooperative but still be able to communicate with the staff.[13] If the indication for sedation is to facilitate an individual medical goal, the sedation level may need to be deeper.[12] The most challenging situation involving sedation arises when the reason for sedation is a humanitarian need. It is here that the greatest variability is seen in the depth of sedation required to provide comfort for a given individual. Sedation for palliative care may range from mild to deep sedation based on the individual desires of the patient and family.[13,14]

The depth of sedation is also individualized and is determined most heavily by the reasons for sedation. The targeted depth of sedation is also determined, in part, by the sedation scales or tools that are used to monitor sedation.[4,13] The more precise the instrument, the more precise the target that can be prescribed. The use of a subjective assessment tool in conjunction with a physiologic assessment tool is thereby indicated to monitor the level of sedation.[15,16] A variety of subjective sedation-assessment tools have been developed and tested with varying degrees of validity and reliability that use some form of numerical reference.[7] Currently the 2 most commonly used are the Richmond Agitation-Sedation Scale (RASS) and the Sedation-Agitation Scale (SAS).[17,18] The 2 most common forms of physiologic sedation-assessment tools are the Bispectral Index (BIS), and the Patient State Index (PSI) monitoring systems.[19,20]

SEDATION CHALLENGES

Achieving and maintaining a specific depth of sedation requires nursing vigilance. Patient response to medication is often unpredictable and varies not only within and between patient populations but also within a single hospital stay for an individual patient. Drug accumulation; changes in hemodynamic status; changes in renal, endocrine, and liver function; and the effects of drug-to-drug interaction can increase or decrease the effectiveness of sedating agents.[12] The challenge of maintaining a specific depth of sedation without incidents of oversedation or undersedation, while allowing the monitoring of a patient's neuroexamination, requires the nurse to be skilled in the art of incorporating both subjective and physiologic data.

In the extremes, undersedation is easy to quantify (patient is awake, patient self-extubates). However, an exact measure of undersedation remains missing from the literature. The 3 reasons for sedation previously cited in this article are injury prevention, facilitation of medical goals, and facilitation of humanitarian goals. Inadequate sedation can lead to decreased patient safety and increased risk of injury. Compromised patient safety as a result of undersedation includes patients removing IV/intra-arterial lines, and unplanned self-extubation.[5] Undersedation can interfere with achievement of medical goals, resulting, for example, in increasing ICP. In addition, end points of palliative care may be compromised with inadequate sedation.

Oversedation is simply stated (more sedation than is required), but is poorly measured. Excessive sedation has been linked to poor outcomes and may result from poorly used or poorly validated scales.[4,20] Oversedation may impair the reliability of the neurologic examination, particularly when the evaluating individual is inexperienced.[16] In contrast with the use of continuous infusions, patients managed with bolus or no sedation have been shown to have significantly higher scores on the SAS (more agitated) and higher BIS scores (more alert) than patients receiving continuous infusions of sedatives/hypnotics.[21] This situation results in higher overall doses of both sedative and analgesic drugs being used in order to achieve the same sedation goals.[4]

Undersedation seems to be less common than oversedation, likely because the adverse effects of undersedation are more dramatic and more rapidly noticed (eg, self-extubation) than the adverse effects of oversedation (eg, immobility). Undersedation contributes to ventilatory asynchrony, patient movement during procedures, and episodes of hemodynamic and intracranial instability in brain-injured individuals.[22] Several studies have examined the incidence of recall of unpleasant events within the critical care setting. However, the SLEAP study investigators[23] concluded that, although recall was common to critical care, there was inadequate evidence to associate sedation interruption and ability to recall events. The researchers suggested that minimizing sedation without undersedation does not increase the risk for recall.

Sedative Use in the Neurocritical Care Unit

Some of the difficulty in optimizing sedation may be attributed to the complexity of drug selection and the drug combinations available, and the practice of allowing broad parameters for nurses when adjusting medication dosages while following a sedation protocol.[24,25] The determination of which sedative to use for neuroinjured patients is not well defined in the literature.[4] A wide variety of medications exists that can be used as sedating agents either singly or in conjunction with other medications.[3,8,26] Central-acting sedatives alter the effects of key neurotransmitters. In the central nervous system (CNS) the major neurotransmitters involved in regulating consciousness are gamma-aminobutyric acid (GABA) and glutamate.[27] GABA is an inhibitory neurotransmitter, and glutamate is an excitatory neurotransmitter.

BENZODIAZEPINES

Benzodiazepines are one of the most common classes of medication used for sedation. Two of the primary benzodiazepines used in the ICU setting are midazolam and lorazepam. Midazolam interacts with receptors in the CNS to increase the inhibitory effect of GABA, which produces an anxiolytic, sedative effect.[28] Lorazepam, like midazolam, globally depresses the CNS function by increasing the effects of GABA but has a longer half-life.[29] Lorazepam is therefore less frequently used because it impedes the ability to quickly and frequently obtain a neuroexamination.

PROPOFOL

Propofol is a phospholipid-based parentally administered anesthetic that is metabolized in the liver and excreted via the kidneys.[30] Propofol inhibits the *N*-methyl-D-aspartate subtype of glutamate receptors by channel gating modulation and has agonistic activity at the GABA receptors. Propofol has a short half-life, which facilitates a shorter time to wake-up for patients who require a neuroexamination as well as shorter time to extubation.[31]

BARBITURATES

Barbiturates, such as pentobarbital and phenobarbital, and opiates, such as morphine and fentanyl, are often used in conjunction with primary-acting sedatives.

Barbiturates, which act as nonselective depressants of the CNS, are capable of producing all levels of CNS mood alteration, ranging from excitation to mild sedation, hypnosis, and deep coma.[32] The sedative-hypnotic and anticonvulsant properties of barbiturates may be related to their ability to enhance and/or mimic the inhibitory synaptic action of GABA, thus interfering with the transmission of excitatory impulses from the thalamus to the cerebral cortex. Hence, barbiturates may be indicated for neurologic patients (eg, seizure prevention or treatment) beyond sedative effect. However, the longer half-life of most barbiturates makes it difficult for nurses to lighten sedation and obtain a neuroexamination at any specific time.

OPIATES

Opiates such as heroin and morphine, derived from the sap of the poppy seed pod, are also often used in conjunction with primary-acting sedatives. Newer agents such as hydromorphone, fentanyl, remifentanil, hydrocodone, and codeine have been pharmacologically synthesized. All of these agents bind to opiate receptors (mu receptors) in the CNS, which results in an inhibition of ascending pain pathways as well as altering pain perception and response to pain. All of the opiates are metabolized in the liver and variably excreted via the kidneys.[33,34]

Hydromorphone is one of the most potent opiate analgesics available and has a half-life of 1 to 3 hours.[32] Heroin is rarely used pharmacologically as an analgesic agent in the United States; however, is legally used in the United Kingdom and a few other countries where it is used to control symptoms of cancer. Heroin has a rapid onset of intense euphoria from high lipid solubility provided by the 2 acetyl groups, resulting in a very rapid penetration of the blood-brain barrier after parenteral administration; in the brain, heroin is then rapidly metabolized into morphine by oxidation of the acetyl groups.[35] However, morphine is a commonly used parenterally applied analgesic agent.[36] In contrast, remifentanil is extremely short acting and cleared by nonspecific esterases located primarily in muscle and intestines.[32] The 2 most commonly used oral analgesics are codeine and hydrocodone. Both of these agents can be used alone or in combination with acetaminophen or aspirin. Codeine is metabolized to morphine. Its duration of action is 4 to 6 hours. Opiates are primarily used as analgesics, but, when used in sufficiently high doses, they may produce a sedationlike side effect and may blunt the neuroexamination.[34]

ALPHA2-ADRENORECEPTOR AGONIST

Dexmedetomidine (Precedex) is increasingly being used for sedation in the critical care setting.[37] Dexmedetomidine is an alpha2-adrenoreceptor agonist with a combination of sedative and analgesic effects.[34] Activation of the alpha2-adrenoreceptor sites within the CNS produces an inhibition in the stress response, thereby facilitating sedation. Dexmedetomidine is administered as a continuous IV infusion not to exceed 24 hours. The elimination half-life is stated as 2 hours.[34]

Although understanding the mechanism of action for various sedatives and analgesics is vital, this knowledge only allows clinicians to ensure that each medication is prescribed and delivered at a correct dosage. The most important decision when choosing a sedative or analgesic agent is to understand what the specific indication for use is at the time the medication is prescribed and what the needs of the patient are at the time.[3–5] If the reason for sedation is facilitating comfort and blunting unpleasant experience, it may be that a longer-acting sedative is indicated. If the patient is acutely critically ill and requires close hemodynamic and physiologic monitoring, then it is likely that the sedation will need to be frequently adjusted and, in the case of obtaining a neuroexamination, interrupted to allow the patient to awaken from the effects of sedation, in which case a shorter-acting agent would be ideal.

THE NEUROLOGIC EXAMINATION

The purpose of serially performed neuroexaminations is to evaluate and track the functional status of the nervous system. The examination requires comprehensively evaluating the patient's level of consciousness (LOC), motor function, sensory function, and cranial nerve reflexes. The combination of ability to open eyes, speak, and follow motor commands constitutes the subcomponents of the Glasgow Coma Score (GCS).[38] The GCS is of great use in monitoring the neurocognitive status of patients with traumatic brain injury. More recently, the Full Outline of Unresponsiveness (FOUR) score has been introduced as a subjective scoring of neurologic injury.[39] The FOUR score evaluates eye response, motor response, brainstem reflexes, and respiratory pattern to provide a score between 0 and 16 (with 16 being a normal response).[40] When used for other conditions, such as spinal cord injury, sedation assessment, or vascular neurologic injury (hemorrhagic and ischemic stroke), the GCS and FOUR score lose specificity and sensitivity as monitoring tools. Because even minor changes in the neuroexamination can have a profound meaning, obtaining a neuroexamination requires that the practitioner is confident that the patient is functioning at the highest possible LOC in order to ensure that the examination results are accurate.[41] Typically, this requires that the examination be done in a sedation-free state; however, because sedation wears off at various ranges, it is not safe to stop a sedative infusion and leave the bedside, nor is it practical to have the nurse stand at the bedside for prolonged periods of time waiting for sedation to wear off.

Changes in the patient's LOC or neurologic level of function can be caused by local anatomic as well as systemic physiologic changes in the brain. Physical changes, such as edema and infarction, cause a dramatic change in the neuroexamination by direct injury to the brain tissue. Chemical changes, such as those seen with narcotics and analgesics, can also cause a dramatic change in the neuroexamination, but these are reversible. Because drugs can impair the validity of the neuroexamination, the examination is most accurate when it is performed in the absence of any sedative effect.

When performing a neurologic examination on a patient who is receiving continuous IV sedation, a nurse is typically instructed to stop the infusion and perform the neuroexamination when the patient is awake. Several problems pertaining to definition arise in determining the construct of awake; what does awake mean and how can clinicians tell? How can clinicians tell when a patient is awake enough to validate the results of a neuroexamination? Do nurse A and nurse B differ in their definitions of awake? Most frequently, the methods of determining when the nurse should obtain the assessment after the sedation has been turned off are:

- Watching for physical cues, such as patient movement
- Watching for cues of wakefulness, such as changing vital signs and spontaneous neurologic function
- Repeating the examination until it is judged to be as good as its going to get
- Using knowledge of the half-life of the sedative agent in use
- Supplementing subjective assessment with physiologic data from a neurofunction monitor

TIMING THE NEUROLOGIC EXAMINATION BASED ON OBSERVATIONAL ASSESSMENT

Physicians and nurses who consistently work at the bedside have highly refined assessment skills and sometimes, with intuition, are able to detect minor changes in patients. However, patients are not all the same and practitioners can be inaccurate. Timing a thorough neurologic examination from subtle cues demands consistent, uninterrupted bedside surveillance and observation for a given set of discrete changes in the patient's condition.[41] Even with a 1:1 nurse/patient ratio, the nurse is not always available at the bedside.[42] Nurses in the ICU setting also vary in their levels of expertise.[43] The ability to interpret subtle cues and changes in patient condition is part of the art of nursing that develops as nurses progress along the continuum from novice to expert. Because novice nurses lack the experience necessary for accurate interpretation of multiple patient cues that signal changes in patient sedation level, they may miss opportunities for appropriately timing the neuroexamination.[44,45]

TIMING THE EXAMINATION BASED ON DRUG HALF-LIFE

Although the effects of many medications, including sedatives, are often described in terms of their half-lives, there are numerous factors that impact rates of metabolism, including hepatic function, renal clearance, and buildup in body fat stores.[34] As such, it is neither practical nor reliable to make a determination of when to perform the neuroexamination based on drug half-life.

TIMING THE EXAMINATION BASED ON HEMODYNAMIC VARIABLES

Often discussed in the clinical setting is a presumed relationship between a patient's hemodynamic response to sedation and the patient's LOC. The most common statement seems to be that an increase in blood pressure and heart rate signal either the presence of pain or the emergence from sedation.[46] However, there are several potential pitfalls with this approach. Changes in heart rate can be attributed to a variety of factors that are not related to emergence from sedation. Hypovolemia, infection, pain, hypotension, hypoxia, and activity, for example, can all contribute to an increase in heart rate. Likewise, an increase in blood pressure may be related to changes in oxygen demand, intravascular fluid volume status, electrolyte concentration, and so forth. A septic patient, for instance, may be receiving a vasopressor to treat septic shock; an increase in blood pressure does not signal emergence from sedation, but is a sign that the vasopressor is effective. A study by Flaishon and colleagues[47] showed a lack of predictive relationship between vital signs and emergence from sedation.

NEUROFUNCTION MONITORING

The 2 primary neurofunction monitors currently available are the BIS monitor and the PSI.[19,20] The BIS monitor was originally developed as an adjunctive tool to be used for assessing a patient's LOC during the intraoperative period. In 2002, BIS monitors were first marketed to the ICU setting. The BIS monitor provides a continuous digital reading of a signal processed single-lead electroencephalogram (EEG) waveform. The BIS scale varies from 0 to 100, with a score of zero corresponding with isoelectric activity and a score of 100 indicating full arousal. The PSI scale also varies from 0 to 100, with zero corresponding with isoelectric activity and 100 indicating full arousal. However, BIS and PSI use different algorithms and are not interchangeable.[48] Hence, the concept that higher BIS or PSI scores correlate with increased levels of arousal, and lower BIS or PSI scores correlate with a lower state of consciousness (more anesthetized).

Neurofunction monitoring has been available for more than 2 decades and is used in the operating room, critical care, outpatient procedures, and even dentistry. Growing evidence now supports the use of BIS monitoring as an adjunct to sedation assessment.[4,16,22,49,50] However, it is important to recognize that this technology is not recommended as a solitary method of sedation assessment and that it should be combined with clinical assessments.[51] Typically, the neurofunction monitor is used for patients receiving continuous IV sedation, with sedation goals being defined jointly in terms of a subjective scale such as the SAS or RASS, and an objective BIS score. This combination of subjective and objective assessment has been associated with a reduced cost of sedation and decreased length of time using mechanical ventilation.[15,22]

RESEARCH SUPPORT FOR NEUROFUNCTION MONITORS AS AN ADJUNCT TO SEDATION ASSESSMENT

Neurofunction monitoring as an adjunct to sedation assessment seems to be indicated for routine use in the critical care setting.[4,16,52–54] Interruptions in sedation are necessary in the neurocritical care setting, but daily interruptions in sedation may not be required in all areas of critical care.[2,55] Recent evidence on daily sedation-vacation protocols has resulted in mixed results regarding the impact of such protocols on length of time using mechanical ventilation and ICU length of stay.[2,13,56]

Staff nurses familiar with BIS or PSI monitoring are at a unique advantage when obtaining a neuroexamination on patients who are receiving continuous IV sedation. Instead of abruptly stopping the IV sedatives, the nurse retains the option to decrease the infusion rate. Once the sedation is decreased, the nurse monitors for an increase in BIS/PSI values. As the BIS values increase, the patient experiences a return to consciousness. Decreasing, instead of stopping, the sedation while observing for an increase in BIS/PSI values may accomplish several goals. First, it allows nurses to incorporate both subjective and objective data into determining when to perform the neuroexamination. Second, it markedly reduces the reliance on nonvalidated subjective clinical assessment parameters. Third, this prevents sudden changes in hemodynamic parameters associated with abruptly stopping sedatives. Fourth, observing the trend in BIS values gives nurses a warning that the patient may be approaching consciousness and ready for a neuroexamination, thereby reducing the risk of causing injury; for example, with an unsafe level of ICP or unplanned self-extubation.

Drug titration does not, and should not, occur solely from a single subjective assessment tool (eg, RASS, or SAS), and nor should drug titration occur solely based on a single physiologic parameter (eg, heart rate, BIS, end-tidal CO_2, or PSI). Instead, the instruments are designed to complement each other. By using the BIS as an adjunct to RASS, nurses avoid the need to repeatedly apply noxious stimuli. Neurofunction monitoring becomes a means of timing when to conduct the neuroexamination. By using technology, nurses are able to have another piece of assessment data. The product of assessment (sum of all assessments) furthers the nurse's knowledge of the patient, which can contribute to accurate interpretation of subtle behaviors during sedation titration.[57] In contrast with timing the neuroexamination based on vital signs, a study by McCann and colleagues[11] showed that BIS scores were a reliable indicator of when the patient will move to command during the emergence from anesthesia for an intraoperative neurologic examination.

LIMITATIONS OF NEUROFUNCTION MONITORING TECHNOLOGY

The BIS and PSI monitors have several limitations that may preclude their use in every patient. For patients with bilateral frontal lobe injury, or patients with trauma in whom there is no space for the sensor, neurofunction monitoring is not practical.

Electromyographic interference from muscle activity can also affect signal-processed EEGs of the BIS monitor. As with any medical technology, clinicians need to determine whether the data represent signal or noise. For example, because muscle contraction produces an electrical signal, BIS and PSI values may be high in a patient who is shivering, even when the patient is fully sedated.

Certain medical therapeutics affect cerebral metabolic activity and may interfere with interpretation of BIS values. One study showed that a decrease in muscle activity (chemical paralysis) was associated with markedly lower BIS values despite the subject being awake.[58] More research is needed to refine the technology to improve practicality in the neurocritical care unit.

SUMMARY

The sedation-assessment conundrum is a result of the conflict created by 2 opposing goals. One goal is to maintain a safe and comfortable environment for patients through sedation. The opposing goal is created by the need to obtain neurologic assessments that reflect the patients' best possible efforts. Planned interruption of continuous IV sedation is a necessary part of the routine nursing practice in neurocritical care. The use of BIS or PSI monitoring as an adjunctive tool for sedation assessment to optimize timing of the neuroexamination in the setting of a planned interruption in sedation is well founded.

Critical care nurses possess the skills and knowledge that allow them to become proficient at incorporating technology into their practice. Sandelowski[57] writes:

> *As the primary machine tenders in health care, nurses often acquire an understanding of how to apply, operate, and interpret the products of devices that become an integral part of the tacit know-how of clinical practice.*

This statement clearly embodies the aspects of critical care that describe the ability of bedside clinicians to understand how and when to place faith in technology, and to find the balance of objective and subjective assessment that will allow them to solve the sedation-assessment conundrum using signal-processed EEG technology in conjunction with acquired subjective assessment skills. Ultimately, best practice embraces using a wide variety of observational and physiologic assessment parameters. Each parameter is not intended to replace the other; instead, a multimodal approach provides a more comprehensive understanding of each patient.[4,59,60]

REFERENCES

1. Olson DM, Graffagnino C, King K, et al. Toward solving the sedation-assessment conundrum: bispectral index monitoring and sedation interruption. Crit Care Nurs Clin North Am 2005;17:257–67.
2. Mehta S, Burry L, Cook D, et al, SLEAP Investigators, Canadian Critical Care Trials Group. Daily sedation interruption in mechanically ventilated critically ill patients cared for with a sedation protocol: a randomized controlled trial. JAMA 2012;308:1985–92.
3. Lacoske J. Sedation options for intubated intensive care unit patients. Crit Care Nurs Clin North Am 2015;27:131–45.
4. Olson DM, Zomorodi MG, James ML, et al. Exploring the impact of augmenting sedation assessment with physiologic monitors. Aust Crit Care 2014;27:145–50.

5. Aitken LM, Bucknall T, Kent B, et al. Sedation protocols to reduce duration of mechanical ventilation in the ICU: a Cochrane Systematic Review. J Adv Nurs 2016; 72:261–72.
6. Sharshar T, Citerio G, Andrews PJ, et al. Neurological examination of critically ill patients: a pragmatic approach. Report of an ESICM expert panel. Intensive Care Med 2014;40:484–95.
7. Olson DM, Thoyre SM, Auyong DB. Perspectives on sedation assessment in critical care. AACN Adv Crit Care 2007;18:380–95.
8. Jacobi J, Fraser GL, Coursin DB, et al. Clinical practice guidelines for the sustained use of sedatives and analgesics in the critically ill adult. Crit Care Med 2002;30:119–41.
9. Dennis LJ, Mayer SA. Diagnosis and management of increased intracranial pressure. Neurol India 2001;49(Suppl 1):S37–50.
10. Alspach J, American Association of Critical-Care Nurses. Core curriculum for critical care nursing. 5th edition. Philadelphia: Saunders; 1998.
11. McCann ME, Brustowicz RM, Bacsik J, et al. The bispectral index and explicit recall during the intraoperative wake-up test for scoliosis surgery. Anesth Analg 2002;94:1474–8, table of contents.
12. Young C, Knudsen N, Hilton A, et al. Sedation in the intensive care unit. Crit Care Med 2000;28:854–66.
13. Burchardi H. Aims of sedation/analgesia. Minerva Anestesiol 2004;70:137–43.
14. Schildmann EK, Schildmann J, Kiesewetter I. Medication and monitoring in palliative sedation therapy: a systematic review and quality assessment of published guidelines. J Pain Symptom Manage 2015;49:734–46.
15. Olson DM, Cheek DJ, Morgenlander JC. The impact of bispectral index monitoring on rates of propofol administration. AACN Clin Issues 2004;15:63–73.
16. Olson DM, Thoyre SM, Peterson ED, et al. Randomized evaluation of bispectral index-augmented sedation assessment in neurological patients. Neurocrit Care 2009;11:20–7.
17. Sessler CN, Gosnell MS, Grap MJ, et al. The Richmond Agitation-Sedation Scale: validity and reliability in adult intensive care unit patients. Am J Respir Crit Care Med 2002;166:1338–44.
18. Riker RR, Picard JT, Fraser GL. Prospective evaluation of the Sedation-Agitation Scale for adult critically ill patients. Crit Care Med 1999;27:1325–9.
19. Riker RR, Fraser GL, Simmons LE, et al. Validating the sedation-agitation scale with the bispectral index and visual analog scale in adult ICU patients after cardiac surgery. Intensive Care Med 2001;27:853–8.
20. Caputo TD, Ramsay MA, Rossmann JA, et al. Evaluation of the SEDline to improve the safety and efficiency of conscious sedation. Proc (Bayl Univ Med Cent) 2011;24:200–4.
21. de Wit M, Epstein SK. Administration of sedatives and level of sedation: comparative evaluation via the Sedation-Agitation Scale and the Bispectral Index. Am J Crit Care 2003;12:343–8.
22. Olson DM, Chioffi SM, Macy GE, et al. Potential benefits of bispectral index monitoring in critical care. A case study. Crit Care Nurse 2003;23:45–52.
23. Burry L, Cook D, Herridge M, et al. Recall of ICU stay in patients managed with a sedation protocol or a sedation protocol with daily interruption. Crit Care Med 2015;43:2180–90.
24. Grap MJ, Munro CL, Wetzel PA, et al. Sedation in adults receiving mechanical ventilation: physiological and comfort outcomes. Am J Crit Care 2012;21: e53–63 [quiz: e64].

25. Skoglund K, Enblad P, Marklund N. Monitoring and sedation differences in the management of severe head injury and subarachnoid hemorrhage among neurocritical care centers. J Neurosci Nurs 2013;45:360–8.
26. Egerod I, Albarran JW, Ring M, et al. Sedation practice in Nordic and non-Nordic ICUs: a European survey. Nurs Crit Care 2013;18:166–75.
27. Bader MK, Littlejohns LR, American Association of Neuroscience Nurses. AANN core curriculum for neuroscience nursing. 5th edition. Glenview (IL): American Association of Neuroscience Nurses; 2010.
28. Bayat A, Arscott G. Continuous intravenous versus bolus parenteral midazolam: a safe technique for conscious sedation in plastic surgery. Br J Plast Surg 2003;56: 272–5.
29. Deem S. Useful information about the pharmacokinetics and pharmacodynamics of midazolam and lorazepam. Anesthesiology 2002;97:522 [author reply: 522–3].
30. Krajcova A, Waldauf P, Andel M, et al. Propofol infusion syndrome: a structured review of experimental studies and 153 published case reports. Crit Care 2015;19:398.
31. Ostermann ME, Keenan SP, Seiferling RA, et al. Sedation in the intensive care unit: a systematic review. JAMA 2000;283:1451–9.
32. Miller RD, Reves JG. Anesthesia. Philadelphia: Churchill Livingstone; 2000.
33. Millgate AG, Pogson BJ, Wilson IW, et al. Analgesia: morphine-pathway block in top1 poppies. Nature 2004;431:413–4.
34. Peck TE, Hill SA. Pharmacology for anaesthesia and intensive care. Cambridge (United Kingdom): Cambridge University Press; 2014.
35. Ford MD. Clinical toxicology. Philadelphia: Saunders; 2001.
36. Aubrun F, Mazoit JX, Riou B. Postoperative intravenous morphine titration. Br J Anaesth 2012;108:193–201.
37. Riker RR, Shehabi Y, Bokesch PM, et al. Dexmedetomidine vs midazolam for sedation of critically ill patients: a randomized trial. JAMA 2009;301:489–99.
38. Teasdale G, Jennett B. Assessment of coma and impaired consciousness. A practical scale. Lancet 1974;2:81–4.
39. Stead LG, Wijdicks EF, Bhagra A, et al. Validation of a new coma scale, the FOUR score, in the emergency department. Neurocrit Care 2009;10:50–4.
40. Wijdicks EF, Bamlet WR, Maramattom BV, et al. Validation of a new coma scale: the FOUR score. Ann Neurol 2005;58:585–93.
41. Olson DM, Graffagnino C. Consciousness, coma, and caring for the brain-injured patient. AACN Clin Issues 2005;16:441–55.
42. Adomat R, Hicks C. Measuring nursing workload in intensive care: an observational study using closed circuit video cameras. J Adv Nurs 2003;42:402–12.
43. Benner P. From novice to expert: excellence and power in clinical nursing practice. Menlo Park (CA): Addison-Wesley Nursing Division; 1984.
44. Rhudy LM, Androwich I. Surveillance as an intervention in the care of stroke patients. J Neurosci Nurs 2013;45:262–71.
45. Hoffman KA, Aitken LM, Duffield C. A comparison of novice and expert nurses' cue collection during clinical decision-making: verbal protocol analysis. Int J Nurs Stud 2009;46:1335–44.
46. Kapoustina O, Echegaray-Benites C, Gelinas C. Fluctuations in vital signs and behavioural responses of brain surgery patients in the intensive care unit: are they valid indicators of pain? J Adv Nurs 2014;70:2562–76.
47. Flaishon R, Windsor A, Sigl J, et al. Recovery of consciousness after thiopental or propofol. Bispectral index and isolated forearm technique. Anesthesiology 1997; 86:613–9.

48. Soehle M, Kuech M, Grube M, et al. Patient state index vs bispectral index as measures of the electroencephalographic effects of propofol. Br J Anaesth 2010;105:172–8.
49. Mondello E, Siliotti R, Noto G, et al. Bispectral Index in ICU: correlation with Ramsay Score on assessment of sedation level. J Clin Monit Comput 2002;17:271–7.
50. Triltsch AE, Welte M, von Homeyer P, et al. Bispectral index-guided sedation with dexmedetomidine in intensive care: a prospective, randomized, double blind, placebo-controlled phase II study. Crit Care Med 2002;30:1007–14.
51. Vivien B, Di Maria S, Ouattara A, et al. Overestimation of Bispectral Index in sedated intensive care unit patients revealed by administration of muscle relaxant. Anesthesiology 2003;99:9–17.
52. Berkenbosch JW, Fichter CR, Tobias JD. The correlation of the bispectral index monitor with clinical sedation scores during mechanical ventilation in the pediatric intensive care unit. Anesth Analg 2002;94:506–11, table of contents.
53. Aneja R, Heard AM, Fletcher JE, et al. Sedation monitoring of children by the Bispectral Index in the pediatric intensive care unit. Pediatr Crit Care Med 2003;4:60–4.
54. Shoushtarian M, Sahinovic MM, Absalom AR, et al. Comparisons of electroencephalographically derived measures of hypnosis and antinociception in response to standardized stimuli during target-controlled propofol-remifentanil anesthesia. Anesth Analg 2016;122:382–92.
55. Schweickert WD, Gehlbach BK, Pohlman AS, et al. Daily interruption of sedative infusions and complications of critical illness in mechanically ventilated patients. Crit Care Med 2004;32:1272–6.
56. MacIntyre NR. Evidence-based ventilator weaning and discontinuation. Respir Care 2004;49:830–6.
57. Sandelowski M. Knowing and forgetting: the challenge of technology for a reflexive practice science of nursing. In: Thorne SE, Hayes VE, editors. Nursing praxis knowledge and action. Thousand Oaks (CA): Sage Publications; 1997. p. 69–85.
58. Messner M, Beese U, Romstock J, et al. The bispectral index declines during neuromuscular block in fully awake persons. Anesth Analg 2003;97:488–91, table of contents.
59. Schneider G, Jordan D, Schwarz G, et al. Monitoring depth of anesthesia utilizing a combination of electroencephalographic and standard measures. Anesthesiology 2014;120:819–28.
60. Le Roux P, Menon DK, Citerio G, et al. Consensus summary statement of the International Multidisciplinary Consensus Conference on Multimodality Monitoring in Neurocritical Care: a statement for healthcare professionals from the Neurocritical Care Society and the European Society of Intensive Care Medicine. Intensive Care Med 2014;40:1189–209.

Obstructive Sleep Apnea and Modifications in Sedation: An Update

Deborah Weatherspoon, PhD, MSN, RN, CRNA[a,*],
Debra Sullivan, PhD, MSN, RN, CNE, COI[b],
Christopher A. Weatherspoon, APRN, MS, FNP-BC[a,c]

KEYWORDS

- Sleep apnea • Obstructive sleep apnea • Sedation

KEY POINTS

- Obstructive sleep apnea is a common medical disorder and unrecognized obstructive sleep apnea may complicate the administration of sedation in the critical care unit.
- A screening tool for obstructive sleep apnea assists critical care nurses to identify patients at increased risk for airway obstruction.
- Sedation should be titrated to achieve comfort without compromise.
- Benzodiazepines should be avoided in patients with obstructive sleep apnea.
- Continuous positive airway pressure or bilevel positive airway pressure may offer needed airway support.

INTRODUCTION

Adequate oxygenation and airway support of patients are always of concern, especially in critical care patients. Many factors contribute to an increased risk for airway compromise and one of the most common contributing factors may be obstructive sleep apnea (OSA). In adults, this disorder is increasingly prevalent,[1] affecting nearly 9% of middle-aged women and 24% of middle-aged men[2]; it is one of the most common medical disorders of sleep.[3] As the name implies, OSA causes reduced or complete airflow disruption during sleep; this in turn reduces oxygenation. Sedation in this

---

This article is an update of an article previously published in *Critical Care Nursing Clinics*, Volume 17, Issue 3, September 2005.

[a] School of Nursing Graduate Program, College of Health Sciences, Walden University, Washington Avenue South, Suite 900, Minneapolis, MN 55401, USA; [b] School of Nursing MSN Program, School of Nursing Graduate Program, College of Health Sciences, Walden University, Washington Avenue South, Suite 900, Minneapolis, MN 55401, USA; [c] Veteran Affairs, Tennessee Valley Health System, Fort Campbell, KY, USA
* Corresponding author.
E-mail address: Deborah.Weatherspoon@Waldenu.edu

Crit Care Nurs Clin N Am 28 (2016) 217–226
http://dx.doi.org/10.1016/j.cnc.2016.02.008 ccnursing.theclinics.com
0899-5885/16/$ – see front matter

population carries an increased risk for hypopnea because it depresses the response to external stimulation and may cause relaxation of pharyngeal muscles during sleep.

Critical care nurses frequently work within titrated ranges of as-needed orders, and must decide on the amount and type of sedation to administer at the point of care. Therefore, it is important for critical nurses to understand OSA and the routinely prescribed sedatives that may affect this disorder. This article provides a basic understanding of the pathophysiology of OSA and traits that may help identify patients with undiagnosed OSA. In addition, the most commonly prescribed sedative pharmacologic agents and adjunctive airway support used in the critical care setting are discussed for use in this population.

ALTERED BREATHING PATTERNS DURING SLEEP

There are 2 types of sleep apnea and either may be of concern for critical care patients. Central sleep apnea (CSA) represents a change in breathing patterns or control, whereas OSA represents abnormal or interrupted air passage caused by obstruction.

Central Sleep Apnea

CSA occurs when the brain fails to transmit adequate signals to the diaphragm and intercostal muscles to initiate ventilation (inhalation). Several conditions may cause CSA, with the most common being associated with congestive heart failure or stroke.

Generally observed during sleep, this breathing pattern presents as a gradual increase and then decrease in breathing effort and airflow. At the weakest point, a total lack of airflow (CSA) may occur. This type of breathing pattern is familiar to most health professionals and is known as Cheyne-Stokes breathing. A formal definition of Cheyne-Stokes breathing is 5 or more central apneas and/or central hypopneas per hour alternating with a crescendo-decrescendo pattern of breathing.[4]

Naughton[5] describes Cheyne-Stokes breathing as a transient, cyclic, or periodic loss of respiratory drive, interspersed with brief periods of hyperventilation. It is usually associated with normal (normocapnia) or low carbon dioxide (CO_2) levels (hypocapnia), measured as $Paco_2$. Certain medications, such as opioids, may also depress the central respiratory center and result in irregular or decreased respiratory patterns (**Box 1**).

Obstructive Sleep Apnea

As the name implies, OSA is a repetitive partial or complete obstruction of the upper airway during sleep.[1] It may be caused by an abnormal anatomic feature or by relaxation of the genioglossus and pharyngeal constrictor muscles causing airway collapse and obstruction. A completely blocked airway without airflow is called an obstructive

Box 1
Conditions associated with CSA

- Congestive heart failure
- Stroke
- Brain injury
- Drug induced: opioids
- Idiopathic CSA

apnea and a partial airway obstruction that results in diminished airflow is called a hypopnea.

A typical cycle of hypopnea and apnea followed by several deep breaths is associated with OSA. The cycle begins as insufficient breathing causes oxygen levels to decrease and CO_2 levels to increase. The body responds by increasing respiratory effort via inspiratory muscles contracting; however, because of the obstruction, there is little or no air movement into the lower airways and lungs. This condition may present as an abdominal rocking motion as the diaphragm descends and increases negative pressure in the thoracic cavity against a closed airway.

As oxygen desaturation progresses and inspiratory effort increases, the person partially, or completely, wakes up gasping for air. Occasionally, patients awaken feeling as if they are choking or smothering. They often move about restlessly, or show twitching of the extremities and then resettle as sleep returns.

A pseudo–Cheyne-Stokes breathing pattern may be observed in patients with OSA. As the airway obstructs and CO_2 level increases, the acute hypercapnia stimulates a compensatory increase in respiratory rate, followed by a return to a slower respiratory rate, then obstruction and apnea. Once the patient awakens enough to improve pharyngeal muscle tone, the cycle begins again (**Table 1**).

IDENTIFYING PATIENTS AT RISK FOR OBSTRUCTIVE SLEEP APNEA

As previously stated, OSA is increasingly common[1] and the condition is underrecognized and often undiagnosed even in symptomatic patients.[6] Increased occurrence rates are seen in middle-aged and older adults. Men are up to 4 times more likely to have OSA, and obesity increases the risk for both genders. A body mass index greater than 30 may increase the risk 7-fold.[6]

Health care providers should be alert for factors that might indicate OSA, beginning with a medical history. The main symptoms of OSA are loud snoring, fatigue, and daytime sleepiness. Patients may be unaware of their own sleep disturbances or snoring and important information is obtained from an immediate family member or bed partner. Fatigue and sleepiness have many causes and are often attributed to overwork and increasing age and recognized as a risk for OSA.

A positive family history of OSA is considered a risk factor and most likely related to anatomic similarities. Numerous genetically influenced or physiologic factors can contribute to upper airway collapse, including anatomic features (eg, craniofacial features), reduced dilator muscle activity during sleep, decreased end-expiratory lung volume, ventilatory control instability, and sleep-state instability, although obesity may outweigh these other predispositions.[7]

Both subjective and objective symptoms may alert clinicians to possible OSA. Patients may report often awakening with a morning headache or a dry mouth, experiencing tiredness or excessive daytime sleepiness, and loss of libido. Objective symptoms include restlessness, snoring loud enough to disturb the patient or others, and recurrent awakening.

Table 1
Comparison of central and OSA

CSA	OSA
Brain fails to initiate regular breathing pattern; loss of respiratory drive	Mechanical obstruction of upper airway
Includes Cheyne-Stokes respiration	May have pseudo–Cheyne-Stokes respiration

Some physical characteristics are easily identified. Inspection of the oropharynx may reveal a large tongue with crowding at the posterior pharynx. A large neck size (>43 cm [17 inches]) or retrognathia (recessed lower jaw) are indicators of increased risk.[6] Obesity and enlarged tonsils increase the likelihood of increased or enlarged mucosal folds. All of these characteristics are associated with crowding of the upper airway and increase the risk of OSA (**Box 2**).

Adults with Down syndrome frequently have OSA, with obstructive apnea, hypoxemia, hypoventilation, and sleep fragmentation.[8] The physical characteristics of Down syndrome, including a large tongue, small nose with flat bridge, and low muscle tone, increase the incidence of OSA in this population. Trois and colleagues[9] measured the occurrence rate and found that 94% of adults with Down syndrome met criteria for OSA.

Comorbid medical conditions may also present clues. Gastroesophageal reflux is a common problem associated with OSA that presents as sudden awakening with dyspnea or choking. A bidirectional association between asthma and OSA has been established in which each disorder negatively influences the other.[10,11]

Untreated OSA is associated with long-term cardiovascular disorders and includes poorly controlled hypertension, heart failure, and cardiac arrhythmias, including atrial fibrillation.[6] Many patients are on antihypertensive drugs, cholesterol medication, and aspirin. High blood pressure, especially if it is resistant to treatment, may indicate a risk for OSA (**Box 3**).

SEDATION IN THE CRITICAL CARE UNIT

Sedation and pain control are important parts of the plan of care for critical care patients. Regardless of the illness or injury that places a patient in the critical care unit (CCU), it can be a frightening experience. In addition, pain is often a factor, whether it is from injury or invasive and unpleasant procedures. Rowe and Fletcher[12] report that agitation frequently occurs in CCU patients.

Sedation decreases the patients' awareness of the environment and reduces their response to stimuli. This therapy is important for critically ill patients because it assists in controlling multiple stress-related symptoms. Sedation varies from light to heavy, depending on the needs of the patient. Heavy sedation is generally needed to facilitate endotracheal tube tolerance and ventilatory support.

PHARMACOLOGIC AGENTS COMMONLY USED IN THE CRITICAL CARE UNIT

Dexmedetomidine hydrochloride (Precedex) is currently a popular choice for sedation in the CCU.[13] Indications and usage include sedation of initially intubated and

Box 2
Symptoms of OSA

- Restless sleep
- Awakening with choking, gasping, or smothering
- Morning headaches, dry mouth, or sore throat
- Waking frequently to urinate
- Awakening unrested, groggy
- Low energy, difficulty concentrating, memory impairment

Box 3
Risk factors for OSA

- Family history
- Increasing age; more common in middle and older age adults
- Male sex; OSA is 2 times more common in men, especially in middle age
- Obesity
- Metabolic syndrome
- Sedation
- Abnormality of the airway: large neck size (>43 cm [17 inches] in men or 41 cm [16 inches] in women), large tongue, retrognathia

mechanically ventilated patients and sedation of nonintubated patients for procedures. One positive for this agent is that patients may be aroused and become alert with stimulation.

Dexmedetomidine does not cause respiratory depression and is useful through the ventilator weaning process. This agent may also be a good choice for early sedation of patients with OSA; however, the dosage and administration should be titrated to the desired clinical effect.

Dexmedetomidine is a selective alpha2-adrenergic agonist with sedative properties. It is administered via intravenous (IV) infusion and is indicated for short-term use. In general, adult sedation in the CCU initiates at 1 μg/kg over 10 minutes, followed by a maintenance infusion of 0.2 to 0.7 μg/kg/h. Patients who are greater than 65 years of age, have hepatic impairment, or are receiving concomitant sedatives, hypnotics, or opioids may require a dose reduction.

Precautions for the administration of dexmedetomidine include continuous monitoring of patients while receiving the sedation. A special-purpose prefilled reservoir device provides an efficient medication delivery system.[14] During a loading dose, transient hypertension may occur and generally does not require treatment.

Young adults with high vagal tone may experience bradycardia or even sinus arrest; this was most evident with rapid IV administration. Treatment includes decreasing or stopping the infusion, administering an anticholinergic such as glycopyrrolate or atropine, or resuscitation as needed. Coadministration with vasodilators or negative chronotropic agents may produce additive pharmacodynamic effects.

Continuous infusion trials of dexmedetomidine for sedation in the CCU setting provide adverse reaction information. One study of 1007 adult patients (17–88 years of age, 43% ≥65 years of age, 77% male, and 93% white) determined adverse reactions.[15] A mean total dose of 7.4 μg/kg (range, 0.8–84.1 μg/kg), mean dose per hour of 0.5 μg/kg/h (range, 0.1–6.0 μg/kg/h), and the mean duration of infusion of 15.9 hours (range, 0.2–157.2 hours) showed that the most frequent adverse reactions were hypotension, bradycardia, and dry mouth.[15]

Prolonged infusion of dexmedetomidine produces a withdrawal syndrome of sympathetic overactivity, characterized by tachycardia, hypertension, and agitation.[16] Long-acting agents, such as oral clonidine, manage the acute withdrawal symptoms.[16]

Propofol

Propofol (Diprivan) is an effective sedative-hypnotic agent with a rapid onset and short half-life used for the induction and maintenance of anesthesia or sedation. Propofol injectable emulsion is a sterile, nonpyrogenic emulsion suitable for IV administration. IV injection of a therapeutic dose of propofol induces hypnosis usually within 40 seconds from the start of injection.[17]

Plasma levels decline rapidly following distribution of a bolus loading dose and a continuous infusion maintains a therapeutic dose. It is typically given as a bolus IV injection of 40 to 100 mg followed by an infusion of 25 to 75 μg/kg/min.[18,19] Decreased doses may be needed in patients greater than 55 years of age (approximately 20 μg/kg/min).[17] Propofol is eliminated by hepatic conjugation to inactive metabolites that are excreted by the kidney. Clearance or the half-life is approximately 1 to 3 minutes and rapid awakening usually occurs within 10 to 15 minutes of discontinuation of infusion. Abrupt discontinuation of propofol may result in rapid awakening with associated anxiety and agitation.

Allergic reactions have been associated with propofol and it is contraindicated in patients with known sensitivity to propofol or allergies to eggs, egg products, soybeans, or soy products. Transient local pain during injection occurs and may be minimized if the larger veins of the forearm or antecubital fossa are used. Pain during IV injection is common and may also be reduced by prior injection of IV lidocaine (1 mL of a 1% solution). Continuous monitoring for early signs of hypotension, apnea, airway obstruction, and/or oxygen desaturation is required.

Pharmacologic advantages of propofol include quick onset and short duration of action, allowing ease of titration and more rapid arousal for weaning and endotracheal extubation.[19] However, propofol lacks analgesic activity, thus requiring adjunctive opioid therapy. Additional adverse effects are reported with long-term use and accumulation in the tissues.[20] More importantly, propofol can cause significant respiratory depression, potentially augmenting the adverse effects of opioid analgesics.[19] The administration of propofol and analgesics in patients with OSA decreases upper airway muscle activity and predisposes these patients to upper airway collapse during inspiration.

BENZODIAZEPINES

Benzodiazepines produce sedation and hypnosis by modulating the main inhibitory neurotransmitter within the central nervous system. Benzodiazepines are administered orally or intravenously as bolus doses or by continuous infusion. There is a growing body of evidence that shows that benzodiazepines are associated with poorer patient outcomes, including increased brain dysfunction, time on mechanical ventilation, and CCU length of stay, and they are not used as commonly as in previous years.

Benzodiazepines are metabolized in the liver. Midazolam has the highest clearance of the benzodiazepines and is most suitable as an infusion (0.04–0.2 mg/kg/hr). Lorazepam has a lower clearance and longer elimination half-life than midazolam. It may be administered as a bolus method of producing sedation (1–4 mg as needed).[13] Diazepam has the lowest clearance of the benzodiazepines and its half-life precludes any common use in the intensive care unit for sedative purposes. It can be given orally (2 mg 3 times daily).[12]

Benzodiazepines may adversely affect the control of ventilation during sleep.[21] The administration of benzodiazepine hypnotics is not recommended in patients with OSA because of potential adverse effects, including a decrease in airway muscle tone and ventilation response to hypoxemia. Flurazepam and midazolam have been reported to increase the severity of OSA and may cause life-threatening conditions for patients with OSA.[22]

OPIOIDS

Opioids provide analgesia, narcosis, and anxiolysis. Often they are combined with sedatives that may produce a synergistic effect. Alone or in combination, opioids should be used with caution for critical patients with OSA. Side effects include respiratory depression, bradycardia, and hypotension secondary to histamine release.

Morphine, hydromorphone, fentanyl, and remifentanil are frequently used opioids in the CCU. Morphine is often given in IV doses of 2 to 5 mg every 5 to 15 minutes until the pain is controlled, followed by similar doses on a scheduled basis every 2 to 4 hours.[18] Renal or hepatic impairment may cause a prolonged effect.

Hydromorphone has a similar, but more potent, analgesia effect. One advantage that hydromorphone has compared with morphine is that it does not cause histamine release and has an improved safety profile in patients with renal disease. A typical IV dosing range is 0.2 to 1.0 mg every 10 to 15 minutes until pain is controlled, followed by similar doses every 2 to 4 hours.[18]

The use of ultrashort remifentanil, a derivative of fentanyl, has increased for several reasons. It is not dependent on hepatic or renal function for metabolism; it has a highly predictable onset and offset, with a short half-life (3–10 min). Remifentanil compared with morphine provided better outcomes for optimal arousal level and necessity of supplemental sedation.[18] In addition, remifentanil and fentanyl have shown equal efficacy in achieving sedation goals.[18]

ALPHA-2 RECEPTOR AGONISTS

Clonidine is useful as an adjunct sedative in the CCU. Clonidine reduces sympathetic outflow, producing profound analgesia and sedation without respiratory depression. It may be administered by bolus doses (50–150 μg every 8 hours) or as an infusion. The addition of clonidine to standard analgesic regimens has been shown to allow reduction of opioid dosage and may facilitate spontaneous respiration. There are some limitations because it may cause an initial increase in arterial pressure followed by a reduction in pressure. In addition, sympathetic and vagal tones are reduced and may lead to bradycardia. Abrupt withdrawal may cause a hypertensive crisis. Clonidine has an elimination half-life of 8.5 hours, which is substantially longer than that of dexmedetomidine, and is metabolized in the liver and excreted into the urine. Dosage adjustment may be necessary and caution is needed in patients with impaired renal function.

Another potential adjunctive sedative agent is ketamine. This *N*-methyl-D-aspartate antagonist protects upper airway patency in patients with OSA while providing dissociative sedation and analgesia without causing upper airway muscle dysfunction.[23] Ketamine has long been established as an effective agent to facilitate ventilator weaning in patients with OSA.[24] Low-dose ketamine was found to decrease agitation and anxiety, manage pain, and prevent respiratory depression in critically ill patients.[25] Although this may be a choice that does not decrease muscle tone and increase risks of OSA, the hemodynamic effects of ketamine may cause concern for myocardial ischemia, increased intracranial pressure, delirium, and sympathetic stimulation.

SURGICAL CRITICAL CARE PATIENTS WITH OBSTRUCTIVE SLEEP APNEA

Patients who have undergone a surgical procedure under general anesthesia are at high risk of a compromised airway, especially in the immediate postanesthesia period. As many as 20% of patients with OSA require a medical intervention related to airway control, including reintubation, in the immediate postoperative period.[3]

Vigilance is necessary and no patient should be left unattended until fully awake. If a patient has a history of OSA, a continuous positive airway pressure (CPAP) machine should be set up and ready for immediate application. Nursing staff assigned to the patient should be thoroughly familiar with potential complications and ready to maintain a difficult airway. In addition, ancillary staff capable of intubating a patient with a difficult airway should be available in-house.

AIRWAY SUPPORT FOR OBSTRUCTIVE SLEEP APNEA IN THE CRITICAL CARE UNIT AND BEYOND

CPAP is a treatment that uses mild air pressure to keep the airways open, and is considered the first-line medical therapy for OSA.[26] A mask that fits securely blows air at a rate that delivers positive pressure from the CPAP machine. Depending on the specific machine, they are quiet and may include options such as heated humidifiers. The mild increased pressure creates an air splint that may prevent the airway collapse that occurs in OSA.

Patients with a prior diagnosis of OSA may have their own CPAP machines that they use at home and be comfortable with this type of airway support. Patients who have never used CPAP may be uncomfortable when first beginning the treatment. Some patients find that exhaling against the continuous pressure is difficult. In these cases, bilevel positive airway pressure (BiPAP) may be a better choice.

BiPAP is similar in function and design to a CPAP machine in that both machine types deliver pressurized air through a mask to the patient's airways. However, BiPAP can be set to include a breath-timing feature that allows a lower pressure for exhalation.[27,28] The air pressure keeps the throat muscles from collapsing and reduces obstructions by acting as a splint. Both CPAP and BiPAP machines allow patients to breathe easily and regularly while sleeping or sedation.

OSA heralds concern for a difficult airway and, in cases in which other airway support does not adequately maintain a patent airway, the laryngeal mask airway (LMA) may be beneficial. The LMA is a tube with a small masklike structure that fits into the oropharynx. This device requires sedation and is most often used for emergency or short-term difficult airway situations.[29]

DISCUSSION

The administration of sedatives, anesthetics, and analgesics in patients with OSA worsens obstruction of the pharynx because of greater depression of the upper airway muscles. With the increase in obesity and the consequent increase in prevalence of OSA, critical care nurses should screen for OSA and be aware of evidence-based guidelines to minimize adverse events related to sedation in critically ill patients. A screening tool known as the Mallampati classification may be used to determine the severity of pharyngeal crowding and risk for OSA.

In addition, nurses should consider that patients in the CCU often present with hemodynamic instability, altered protein binding, and impaired organ function that creates unpredictable pharmacokinetics and pharmacodynamics,[18] which increases the difficulty of achieving benefit from analgesic and sedative medications without harm from their associated complications.

Balancing the type and amount of sedation is possible; however, it requires an attentive approach unique to each patient. Finding the combination and amount necessary to achieve a desirable outcome rests on the critical care nurse who is continuously assessing and monitoring the patient. In patients with OSA, sedation may interfere with the ability to awaken from sleep and can lengthen periods of apnea, with potentially dangerous consequences. Even patients with a secure endotracheal airway require a careful balance of sedation in order to tolerate the endotracheal tube without interfering with ventilator weaning.

SUMMARY

This article presents the background and basic physiology of sleep disorders that affect respiration, with a focus on OSA. Physical characteristics of patients at risk for airway obstruction provide nurses with needed information to identify and take added precautions with these patients. The importance of sedation, pain, and airway control in patients with OSA is emphasized. The most commonly used sedative and analgesic pharmacologic agents and adjunctive airway support mechanisms are discussed to assist critical care nurses in planning care for this at-risk population.

REFERENCES

1. Peppard PE, Young T, Barnet JH, et al. Increased prevalence of sleep-disordered breathing in adults. Am J Epidemiol 2013;177:1006–14.
2. Gottlieb DJ, Punjab NM, Mehra R, et al. CPAP versus oxygen in obstructive sleep apnea. N Engl J Med 2014;370:2276–85.
3. Venn JH. Obstructive sleep apnea and anaesthesia. Anaesth Intensive Care Med 2011;12:7.
4. Berry RB, Budhiraja R, Gottlieb DJ, et al. Rules for scoring respiratory events in sleep: update of the 2007 AASM Manual for the Scoring of Sleep and Associated Events. Deliberations of the Sleep Apnea Definitions Task Force of the American Academy of Sleep Medicine. J Clin Sleep Med 2012;8(5):597–619.
5. Naughton MT. Cheyne-Stokes respiration. Sleep Med Clin 2014;9(1):13–25.
6. Kingman P, Strohl MD. Obstructive sleep apnea. Merck Manuals professional edition. Available at: http://www.merckmanuals.com/professional/pulmonary-disorders/sleep-apnea/obstructive-sleep-apnea. Accessed March 1, 2016.
7. Sehgal A, Mignot E. Genetics of sleep and sleep disorders. Cell 2011;146:194–207.
8. Capone GT, Aidikoff JM, Taylor K, et al. Adolescents and young adults with Down syndrome presenting to a medical clinic with depression: co-morbid obstructive sleep apnea. Am J Med Genet 2013;161:2188–96.
9. Trois MS, Capone GT, Lutz JA, et al. Obstructive sleep apnea in adults with Down syndrome. J Clin Sleep Med 2009;5(4):317–23.
10. Teodorescu M, Plomis DA, Hall SV, et al. Association of obstructive sleep apnea risk with asthma control in adults. Chest 2010;138(3):543–50.
11. Teodorescu M, Barnet JH, Hagen EW, et al. Association between asthma and risk of developing obstructive sleep apnea. JAMA 2015;313(2):156–64.
12. Rowe K, Fletcher S. Sedation in the intensive care unit. Cont Educ Anaesth Crit Care Pain 2008;8(2):50–5.
13. Kemp KM, Henderlight LT, Nevilee MW. Precedex: is it the future of cooperative sedation? Nursing 2008;38:7–8.
14. Kriesel MS, Kriesel JW, Thompson TW. Special purpose fluid dispenser. US patent; 2012. Available at: file:///C:/Users/dweatherspoon/Downloads/US8287521.pdf. Accessed March 1, 2016.
15. Precedex-Hospira. Highlights of prescribing information. Available at: https://www.hospira.com/en/images/EN-4003_tcm81-92504.pdf. Accessed March 1, 2016.

16. Kukoyi AT, Coker SA, Lewis LD, et al. Two cases of acute dexmedetomidine withdrawal syndrome following prolonged infusion in the intensive care unit: report of cases and review of the literature. Hum Exp Toxicol 2013;32(1):107–10.
17. Food and Drug Administration. Diprivan (propofol) injectable emulsion. Available at: http://www.accessdata.fda.gov/drugsatfda_docs/label/2008/019627s046lbl.pdf Accessed March 1, 2016.
18. Hughes CG, McGrane S, Pandharipande PP. Sedation in the intensive care setting. Clin Pharmacol 2012;4:53–63.
19. Thoma BN, Li J, McDaniel CM, et al. Clinical and economic impact of substituting dexmedetomidine for propofol due to a US drug shortage: examination of coronary artery bypass graft patients at an urban medical centre. Pharmacoeconomics 2014;32(2):149–57.
20. Jakob SM, Ruokonen E, Grounds M, et al. Dexmedetomidine vs midazolam or propofol for sedation during prolonged mechanical ventilation: two randomized controlled trials. JAMA 2012;307:1151–60.
21. Gonçalves M, Oliveira A, Leao A, et al. The impact of benzodiazepine use in nocturnal O2 saturation of OSAS patients. Sleep Med 2013;14:e141–2.
22. Zhang XJ, Li QY, Wang Y, et al. The effect of non-benzodiazepine hypnotics on sleep quality and severity in patients with OSA: a meta-analysis. Sleep Breath 2014;18(4):781–9.
23. Ankichetty S, Wong J, Chung F. A systematic review of the effects of sedatives and anesthetics in patients with obstructive sleep apnea. J Anaesthesiol Clin Pharmacol 2011;27(4):447–58.
24. Brown DL. Use of ketamine to wean a patient with sleep apnea. Crit Care Med 1986;14(2):167–8.
25. Moitra VK, Patel MK, Darrah D, et al. Low-dose ketamine in chronic critical illness. J Intensive Care Med 2016;31(3):216–20.
26. Jordan AS, McSharry DG, Malhotra A. Adult obstructive sleep apnoea. Lancet 2014;383(9918):736.
27. Blau A, Minx M, Peter JG, et al. Auto bi-level pressure relief–PAP is as effective as CPAP in OSA patients—a pilot study. Sleep Breath 2012;16(3):773–9.
28. Johnson KG, Johnson DC. Treatment of sleep-disordered breathing with positive airway pressure devices: technology update. Med Devices (Auckl) 2015;8: 425–37.
29. Ghaus MS. Laryngeal Mask Airway Supreme™ for difficult airway management and establishing ventilation in the intensive care unit. Indian J Anaesth 2014; 58(1):91–3.

Complications of Sedation in Critical Illness: An Update

Jan Foster, PhD, APRN, CNS

KEYWORDS

- Sedation • Complications • Post-ICU syndrome • ICU-acquired weakness • Costs

KEY POINTS

- Oversedation is associated with short- and long-term complications, namely post–ICU syndrome (PICS), and excessive costs.
- Management and prevention of complications are most successful with a collaborative, team approach, using research-based strategies.
- Assessment of sedation level and muscle strength with valid and reliable instruments promotes communication, care planning, and early intervention that reduces the risk of long-term complications of sedation.

INTRODUCTION

In the mid-1990s Dave, a 41-year-old otherwise healthy man, presented to the emergency department of a small community hospital with shortness of breath and altered mental status. He was placed on a nonrebreather oxygen mask, but with increasing hypoxemia and dyspnea was intubated and placed on mechanical ventilator support with maximum settings. He was diagnosed with community-acquired pneumonia and sepsis; over the next several weeks he developed acute respiratory distress syndrome (ARDS), empyema, and sinusitis. Management was complicated by allergy to sensitive antibiotics, along with nicotine and opiate withdrawal, which he took for chronic cervical neck and back pain from an earlier injury. Agitation, high fevers, and tachycardia remained for days, despite heavy doses of lorazepam, propofol, and occasional doses of cisatracurium or pancuronium to facilitate work of breathing. Three weeks later Dave was weaned from sedation and extubated. This was not, however, the end of his medical problems.

Dave experienced extreme muscle wasting, leaving him very weak and unstable during ambulation attempts. He also reported disturbed sleep patterns with frequent

This article is an update of an article previously published in Critical Care Nursing Clinics, Volume 17, Issue 3, September 2005.
No conflicts of interest to report.
Nursing Inquiry & Intervention, Inc, The Woodlands, TX 77381, USA
E-mail address: jgwfoster@comcast.net

Crit Care Nurs Clin N Am 28 (2016) 227–239
http://dx.doi.org/10.1016/j.cnc.2016.02.003 ccnursing.theclinics.com
0899-5885/16/$ – see front matter

bizarre dreams during and following sedation administration, leaving him so fatigued it interfered with pulmonary and physical rehabilitation during the day. Focal weakness in his right leg became apparent, along with foot drop. Electromyography and nerve conduction studies demonstrated a peroneal nerve injury. Physical therapy was initiated in the acute care hospital and continued in a rehabilitation facility following discharge. Years later, impaired dorsiflexion interfered with safe operation of a motor vehicle and Dave was rendered unable to drive.

Although use of sedation is a necessary component of care for the critically ill, careful and vigilant monitoring to guard against oversedation, with frequent sedation holiday attempts, is necessary to prevent complications not only in the acute care setting but also to minimize long-term problems, delayed return to functional status, and jeopardized quality of life following critical illness. Despite prudent use of sedatives and neuromuscular blocking agents, with dosing guided by a sedation scale and peripheral nerve monitoring, respectively, parenteral and enteral nutrition, and physical therapy, Dave suffered some of the long-term sequelae of critical illness, heavy sedation, and neuromuscular blockade frequently reported in the literature.

Two decades later, this constellation of deficits, among others, has been termed post–intensive care syndrome (PICS).[1] Cumulative data of intensive care unit (ICU) admissions, discharges, mortality, and survivorship indicate that in the United States, nearly 6 million patients are admitted to ICU annually, with approximately 5 million survivors discharged.[2] Although they have survived the critical illness, long-term deficits in pulmonary, neuromuscular, and physical function remain. Psychiatric symptoms and cognitive impairment may develop and/or persist; these problems in turn lead to compromises in quality of life for survivors and family members.[3]

POST–INTENSIVE CARE SYNDROME

Pulmonary Complications

Pulmonary complications following critical illness are documented predominately in patients who had ARDS. Most studies have been conducted within 6 to 12 months following ICU discharge; however, one study occurred with a median follow-up time of 5.5 years. At least one abnormal pulmonary function test was present in 27 of 50 patients (54%) who had ARDS; the most common impairment was a restriction in forced expiratory volume in 1 second/forced vital capacity ratio, found in 16 patients.[4] This is a measure of the proportion of vital capacity able to be expired in the first second of a forced expiration; it indicates that obstructive lung condition persisted following ARDS. The researchers also found that patients with abnormalities in multiple pulmonary function tests (diffusion capacity and total lung capacity) reported significantly lower health-related quality of life, measured by Short Form-36 scores.[4]

Neuromuscular Complications

An estimated 50% of ICU patients have severe weakness during critical illness that persists for months or even years.[5,6] Critically ill individuals have multiple reasons for the development of skeletal muscle weakness, stemming from neuropathophysiologic and myopathic abnormalities. Although there have been some conflicting results, studies have identified local and systemic inflammatory mediator release during sepsis and other severe insult, multiorgan dysfunction, ARDS, prolonged ventilator dependence, corticosteroid use, neuromuscular blockade, hyperglycemia, and immobility and disuse atrophy as causes for neuromuscular dysfunction in the critically ill.[5–7]

Critical illness polyneuropathy (CIP) has been described in the literature for more than three decades. It is characterized by severe weakness in proximal and distal muscles of the extremities, deep tendon arreflexia, and diaphragmatic weakness that may interfere with ventilator weaning.[8] Sensory nerve findings include loss of pain, temperature, and vibration sensation distally, although with nonresponsive patients this may be difficult to determine. Electrodiagnostic studies show evidence of diffuse axonal degeneration of peripheral nerves. There is absence of decremental response to repetitive nerve stimulation, decreased amplitude in sensory nerve action potentials in two or more nerves, decreased amplitude in compound muscle action potentials in two or more nerves, and normal conduction velocity.[9,10] In one of the earlier studies, Fletcher and associates[11] found motor or sensory deficits in 59% of 22 patients studied. Twenty-one had electromyographic indications of chronic partial denervation associated with axonal neuropathy. They concluded that CIP causing extreme weakness can last for 5 years after critical illness.

Critical illness myopathy (CIM) has also been identified as a source of persistent severe weakness in the critically ill. It often coexists with CIP and may be difficult to distinguish the two. It also is linked with sepsis, multiorgan dysfunction, and mechanical ventilation; and female gender and steroid use.[12] CIM is suspected by clinical presentation of extreme muscle weakness and more conclusively determined by direct muscle stimulation during electrophysiology studies and muscle biopsy. Electromyography requires awake patients who can contract muscle on command, which cannot always be accomplished in the critically ill. When electrodiagnostics are possible, findings include decreased muscle membrane excitability in two or more muscle groups with direct muscle stimulation, low amplitude motor unit potentials with early or normal full recruitment with or without fibrillation potentials using needle electromyogram in two or more muscle groups, and normal to near-normal sensory nerve action potentials, which aids in discriminating from CIP.[10] Muscle biopsy results show multiple pathologic findings that include acute necrosis, atrophy of type II (fast twitch) fibers, and thick filament (myosin) loss.[9] Because it is an invasive procedure, lacks priority in the presence of critical illness, and findings may not be immediately available, muscle biopsy is often impractical in the ICU.

Use of neuromuscular blocking agents for ARDS and ventilator management, intracranial pressure control, protection of delicate microvascular surgery, and so forth proliferated during the 1980s and 1990s. Persistent paralysis and severe weakness following termination of neuromuscular blockade prompted increased research in neuromuscular dysfunction. Some patients exhibit elements of both CIP and CIM. Eighteen different terms for ICU muscle weakness appeared in the literature.[10] This, along with lack of diagnostics and clarity around an explanation for severe and prolonged weakness, further complicated the issue for researchers and clinicians. In some research reports, diagnostic criteria have lacked uniformity and in others, failed to clearly differentiate the two phenomena. Increasingly, the term critical illness neuromyopathy (CINM) has come to be used in clinical practice and in research. Articulating and communicating the patient's condition in the clinical setting has been problematic, which in turn complicates a plan for prevention and management. Hence, the condition frequently goes unnoticed. The term ICU-acquired weakness (ICUAW)[10,13] has been proposed and comes with this definition[10]:

> *ICUAW designates clinically detected weakness in critically ill patients in whom there is no plausible etiology other than critical illness. Three subcategories are included: CIP designates patients with electrophysiological evidence of axonal polyneuropathy; CIM denotes patients with electrophysiological and/or histological evidence of myopathy; CINM indicates patients with coexisting electrophysiological and/or histological evidence of CIP and CIM.*

This helps to solve the either/and/or argument regarding CIP, CIM, or CINM and the focus can then move on to the larger issues of recognizing ICUAW in the clinical setting, and facilitating research on the subject.

Disuse Atrophy

Disuse atrophy is another neuromuscular complication of PICS. Prolonged bedrest and immobility associated with sedative use in critically ill patients induces severe muscle inactivity, followed by disuse atrophy, leading to further impairment of physical mobility in cyclical fashion. Skeletal muscle atrophy can begin within 4 hours of inactivity, with damage worsening as activity limitations persist.[14] Cellular mechanisms, signaling, and feedback processes during normal activity that regulate protein synthesis, degradation, and programmed death are disrupted during periods of inactivity.[15] Two chief mechanisms underlie muscle atrophy stemming from inactivity during critical illness: a decrease in protein synthesis and an increase in muscle degradation. During bedrest and inactivity, muscles are subjected to lower mechanical loads and sustained for shorter periods. Over time, this decrease in force and power output (mechanical unloading) triggers catabolism of muscle and dampens contractility, resulting in smaller, weaker muscles. Apoptosis, which is regulated cell death, also occurs with mechanical unloading and contributes to muscle atrophy.[15] A decrease in muscle mass, muscle fiber diameter, and number of fibers per muscle results. Changes at the cellular level include rupture of the sarcolemmel membrane, streaming of Z bands, and split sarcomeres.[14]

Sedation is indirectly associated with ICUAW and disuse atrophy. Of multiple covariates, prolonged mechanical ventilation has been directly linked to ICUAW.[6] Although practice has changed in recent years, sedatives continue to be a mainstay of ventilator management. Early on, heavy sedation was necessary to blunt patient breathing efforts because the ventilators were rigid in volume and insensitive to patient initiation of breaths. Developments in ventilator technology, along with recognition that patients do better with less sedation, has led to such practices as intermittent dosing versus continuous infusion and daily sedation holiday. However, any sedation for ventilator management or other purposes renders patients immobile or with reduced mobility at best. Sedatives hinder activity and movement, with increasing loss of muscle contraction for posture, weight bearing, and resistance to gravity. Muscles increasingly weaken and shrink in size, hence the progression of disuse atrophy with sedative use.

Physical Function Complications

Impairments in physical function reportedly occur in more than 50% of patients as far out as 1 year after ICU discharge.[16] In a study of 1738 patients admitted to ICU, health-related functional status and the impact of sickness was measured in 255 respondents 1 year following discharge with the Sickness Impact Profile-68. Greatest dysfunction was found in mobility control and social behavior, indicated by frequently cited illustrations of poor function. Examples include the following[16]:

- I am not doing heavy work around the house
- I walk more slowly; shorter distances; stop often to rest
- My sexual activity has decreased
- I am doing fewer community activities

In an earlier quality-improvement study to evaluate disposition and condition of patients discharged from the hospital, project leaders reported that 5% to 20% of patients conveyed they had a high degree of disability and 11% to 33% of patients had partial disability 1 year following discharge. Additionally, 12% to 23% required complete assistance with activities of daily living with 25% to 55% requiring some assistance.[17] Walking, sexual activity, social interaction, and activities of daily living require sufficient energy, muscle integrity, and strength. As demonstrated in these studies, the deconditioning that occurs in the ICU, exacerbated by overzealous use of sedation and consequent immobility, clearly has lasting effects on various aspects of physical function.

Psychiatric Complications

Survivors of critical illness reportedly experience depression, anxiety, and posttraumatic stress disorder (PTSD) long after ICU discharge,[3] with depression the most commonly occurring disorder.[18] Three months after general medical-surgical patients with respiratory failure or shock were discharged from the hospital, 37% (149 out of 407 respondents) reported depressive symptoms; also 12 months after hospital discharge, 33% (116 of 347) reported depressive symptoms, using the Beck Depression Inventory–II scale.[18,19] These findings are similar to an earlier systematic review of general ICU patients in which a median of 28% of patients reported depressive symptoms[20] and in another systematic review of patients surviving ARDS, 17% to 43% of 277 patients with a median of 28% reporting symptoms of depression. Follow-up times varied among the six studies included in the review, ranging from immediately after discharge to 12, 19, 24, 48, 57, and 96 months.[21] Anxiety occurred in 23% to 48% of 208 survivors, with a median of 24%.[21]

PTSD has been increasingly associated with survival of critical illness. In a study of 255 patients, van der Schaaf and colleagues[16] found that 18% reported symptoms of PTSD 1 year after ICU discharge. Jackson and colleagues[18] reported lower numbers, with 7% (27 of 415 and 24 of 361) of patients reporting symptoms of PTSD at 3 and 12 month follow-up times, respectively. These differences could be explained by the use of different criteria or scales for measurement: Impact of Events Scale[22] versus the Post–Traumatic Stress Checklist–Specific Version of the Diagnostic and Statistical Manual-IV.[23] Among other factors, use of sedatives during the ICU stay has been associated with these psychiatric symptoms.

Cognitive Complications

Memory impairment, attention deficit, delirium, and loss of general cognitive processing are common during and after critical illness.[3] Multiple factors are associated with cognitive dysfunction, demonstrated in various studies over the years. Sedative use has been linked to delirium in several investigations; in an early study, lorazepam was one of 11 covariates shown to be an independent risk factor for onset of delirium in the ICU.[24] Midazolam also contributes to risk for delirium, especially when given as a continuous infusion versus intermittent boluses (odds ratio, 1.04; 95% confidence interval, 1.03–1.06/odds ratio, 0.97; 95% confidence interval, 0.88–1.05, respectively).[25] Cognitive dysfunction can be long-lasting. Even when sedatives are interrupted on a daily basis for spontaneous awakening and breathing trials, cognitive impairment has been observed at 3- and 12-month intervals.[26]

Quality of Life

The pulmonary, neuromuscular, physical, psychiatric, and cognitive difficulties of PICS contribute to compromises in overall quality of life. Much deterioration in quality of life relates to poor physical function, with some improvements within a year after ICU discharge. However, this may not be sustainable. In a longitudinal study of 300 patients, most had achieved significant recovery within 1 year of ICU discharge but experienced a subsequent decline 2.5 to 5 years out.[27] Survivors may not be able to return to employment, which can have serious financial implications; assume family roles, interfering with self-esteem; or participate in social functions as they did before their critical illness. These consequences in turn further diminish quality of life. With 5 million survivors of critical illness in the United States, clearly there are thousands of individuals living in the community with life-changing physical and psychological impairment.

COST FACTORS OF SEDATION

There are several ways to look at the costs of sedation use in ICU. First is the off-the-shelf or acquisition cost of the drug. This is the "price tag" placed on the medication, generally by the pharmacy service or department, which is often negotiated according to volume used by the hospital. Dispensation of medications to patients and consequential pricing comes from the pharmacy budget; for this reason, the pharmacy department (and/or pharmacists) may discourage use of "expensive" drugs. However, "cheaper" drugs may induce complications, such as prolonged recovery times after cessation of the drug. Extended ventilator dependence, ICU stay, and hospital stay may result. Generally the ICU or other medical services bear this cost. This is the real cost to the hospital, however, or for participants in an Accountable Care Organization, by the hospital system because patients move from the acute care facility to the long-term acute care facility.

Studies evaluating the pharmacoeconomics of sedative use in the ICU are largely focused on cost avoidance associated with choice of sedative that results in fewer ventilator days and shorter ICU length of stay. For example, Bioc and colleagues[28] compared the costs of dexemedetomidine or propofol with lorazepam or midazolam and determined that the weighted cost of the medication per patient was much lower for the benzodiazepine group ($65) versus the nonbenzodiazepine group ($1327). However, the overall ICU cost for the benzodiazepine group was much higher at $45,394 compared with $35,380 for the nonbenzodiazepine group. The investigators ascribed the higher costs for the benzodiazepine group to more days using mechanical ventilation, with 6.3 days mean time for this group versus 4.3 days for the nonbenzodiazepine group. Also, the mean time to discharge for the benzodiazepine group was 11.5 compared with 8.3 days for the nonbenzodiazepine group.[28] These findings were consistent with six studies included in a systematic review in which there were fewer ventilator days and shorter ICU stays when nonbenzodiazepines were administered instead of midazolam or lorazepam; however, no cost data were reported.[29]

Second are the costs to the patients and the potential long-term complications associated with excessive doses and/or duration of the medications. Severe weakness and physical and cognitive dysfunction may cost the individual his or her job, with resulting financial difficulties for survivors and their families. Add to that the costs of the hospitalization, rehabilitation, and follow-up care and the financial liability can be astronomical.

Finally, there are societal costs, which may be two-fold. Most obvious of these is loss of income during periods of unemployment, which may become permanent, resulting in fewer tax dollars funneled into the system. With a potential for increased dependence on public funding, the net result is the survivor consumes more than he or she contributes. Loss of employment may not only impose a monetary burden on society but there is also loss of the survivor's contributions in talent, skill, and other valued assets.

PREVENTING COMPLICATIONS OF SEDATION

Appropriate use of sedation to prevent complications is a multidimensional problem; clinicians and researchers must look for solutions in a variety of places. Assessment of sedation with a combination of instruments, selection of the appropriate medication and method of delivery, and an individualized plan are tools currently available to best meet patients' needs.

Measuring Level of Sedation

Appropriate sedation begins with assessment for and management of underlying causes of agitation, such as pain, anxiety, hypoxemia, fever, and withdrawal syndromes. Next, care providers must communicate the goals of sedation. The critical care team must agree on end points of adequate sedation and use the same measures of assessment. More than 30 subjective scales for measurement of sedation level have been described in the medical literature.[30] Formal evaluation for reliability and validity is reported, however, in only 12 adult dedicated instruments: the Ramsay,[31] Observer's Assessment of Alert/Sedation Scale,[32] Harris Scale,[33,34] Sheffield Sedation Scale,[35] Motor Activity Assessment,[36] Vancouver Interaction and Calmness Scale,[37] Sedation-Agitation Scale,[38] Richmond Agitation-Sedation Scale,[39] Adaptation to the Intensive Care Environment,[40] Minnesota Sedation Assessment,[41] Sedation Intensive Care Score,[42] and Nursing Instrument for the Communication of Sedation.[43]

In a systematic review of the literature, Robinson and colleagues[44] further evaluated the use of these scales by categorizing them according to strength of psychometric properties, using a 20-point scoring system. They concluded that only two scales achieved a "very good" status, six were rated as having "moderate" properties, and two were rated as having "very low" properties. Much work has been done on validation of sedation assessment and scoring systems since Dave's critical illness in the 1990s; clinicians are urged to select the best valid and reliable scale suited to their patient population and most accepted among team members. In so doing, communication and achievement of patient-centered goals is optimized (**Table 1**).

Sedative Choice and Administration Strategies

Since the mid-1990s, there has been vast knowledge growth about sedative use and delivery approach for potentially diminishing complications. The days of "keeping patients quiet" are now taboo, with increased recognition of the importance of allowing patients mobility and interaction with the environment. For example, benzodiazepine use has been associated with delirium onset in the ICU.[24,25] Clinicians are urged to limit use of these drugs or when unavoidable, to use smaller dosing amounts. In a study of ICU patients receiving midazolam, patients were more likely to develop

Table 1
Sedation assessment scales and strength of psychometric properties

Very Good	Moderate	Very Low
Richmond Agitation-Sedation Scale	Vancouver Interaction and Calmness Scale	Sheffield Sedation Scale
Sedation-Agitation Scale	Adaptation to the Intensive Care Environment	Observer's Assessment of Alertness/Sedation Scale
	Ramsay Sedation Scale	
	Minnesota Sedation Assessment Tool	
	Nursing Instrument for the Communication of Sedation	

Adapted from Robinson BR, Berube M, Barr J, et al. Psychometric analysis of subjective sedation scales in critically ill adults. Crit Care Med 2013;41(9 Suppl 1):S16–29.

delirium with a continuous infusion than with intermittent boluses,[25] which could be attributed to a lower cumulative dose.

Alternative sedative selection may be effective in deterring some immediate and long-term complications of sedation. Krupp and Balas describe the clinical practice guidelines for pain, agitation, and delirium, and provide suggestions for nonbenzodiazepine sedatives, along with some of the advantages (see Krupp A, Balas MC: Application of Clinical Practice Guidelines for Pain, Agitation, and Delirium, in this issue). Weatherspoon and coworkers provide recommendations for alternative sedatives, along with detailed prescribing information (see Weatherspoon D, Sullivan D, Weatherspoon CA: Obstructive Sleep Apnea and Modifications in Sedation – An Update, in this issue).

Daily sedation holiday is another tactic for limiting complications of sedation. In an earlier study, Kress and colleagues found that ventilator days were reduced from 7.3 to 4.9 days ($P = .004$) and ICU length of stay was decreased from 9.9 to 6.4 days ($P = .02$) when sedatives (propofol or midazolam and morphine) were interrupted on a daily basis.[45] Sedation holiday has since become a component of the ABCDE Bundle. When coordinated awakening and breathing trials were implemented with other elements of the Bundle, delirium monitoring/management and early mobility, Balas and colleagues[46] found a significant reduction in delirium compared with patients who did not participate in the Bundle (odds ratio, 0.55; 95% confidence interval, 0.33–0.93; $P = .03$); and increased the likelihood of moving out of bed (odds ratio, 2.11; 95% confidence interval, 1.29–3.45; $P = .003$). Sedation holiday has become a widespread practice, with many ICU teams showing encouraging results through quality improvement and evidence-based practice projects, sharing their successes at professional meetings and in digital and print publications.

Light versus deep sedation may be an effective strategy for better ICU outcomes after discharge. Treggiari and colleagues[47] found that when patients were maintained at a Ramsay sedation score level of 1 (awake and anxious, agitated, or restless) or 2 (awake, cooperative, oriented, tranquil) they were liberated from mechanical ventilation on average 1 day sooner compared with patients who were deeply sedated with Ramsay scores of 3 (awake, responds only to commands) or 4 (asleep with brisk response to light touch or loud noise). Additionally, at 1 month following discharge patients in the deep sedation group experienced more PTSD ($P = .07$), greater problems with memory ($P = .02$), and more disturbing memories ($P = .05$).[47] Also, there were no adverse events in the light sedation group, which has troubled critical care nurses over the years, with legitimate concerns regarding such issues as self-extubation, tachycardia, or hypertension. Aside from the benefits to mental health, fewer days using mechanical ventilation carries the benefit of patients receiving less sedation for ventilator tolerance and shorter periods of immobility.

Assessing Muscle Strength and Activity

Knowing that sedative use in critically ill patients induces limited mobility even with light sedation, leading to skeletal muscle weakness, atrophy, and further inactivity, vigilant assessment and early intervention may help to disrupt this cycle. The Medical Research Council (MRC) muscle strength scoring system is a validated instrument useful in assessing progressive weakness. The basic scoring method is familiar to many if not all critical care nurses; muscle strength ranges from 0 (no movement or contraction) to 5 (fully normal strength).[48] In assessing ICUAW, a comprehensive score is derived from assessment of three muscle groups in the upper extremities (upper arm abductors, elbow flexors, wrist extensors) and three in the lower extremities (hip flexors, knee extensors, and foot dorsal flexors) in bilateral fashion, with a highest possible score of 60. A score of less than 48 is consistent with significant weakness.[12]

A drawback to the MRC scale is that it requires intact level of consciousness and awareness in order for the individual to follow instructions when testing volitional movement against gravity and resistance. Because critically ill individuals often have altered consciousness as a result of their illness or injury, presence of delirium, or because of administration of sedatives, the muscle scoring system may not accurately reflect muscle integrity (**Box 1**).

Another method of muscle strength assessment that holds promise is with use of handgrip dynamometry. The instrument provides a quantifiable measure of strength that is compared with standardized values; a normal range for men is 101 to 121 pounds force and for women the range is 57 to 70 pounds force. Three readings for each hand are averaged and recorded; the test can be repeated daily allowing for comparisons over time.[49] Advantages to handgrip dynamometry assessment of muscle strength include greater objectivity with quantifiable results, less disruption to patients, and increased efficiency for nurses by testing fewer muscle groups. However, as with the MRC, patients must be attentive enough to follow instructions. Whenever and as soon as possible in the ICU stay, muscle strength evaluation should be incorporated into the daily or shift assessment so that interventions can be initiated to minimize muscle weakness and atrophy.

Early mobility is a well-supported strategy for improving patient well-being while in the ICU and preventing some of the long-term complications of oversedation. Mobilizing patients even while intubated with intravenous catheters and other devices that typically encumber ICU patients is feasible and does not increase risk for harm. Early, protocolized mobility results in fewer days on bedrest, and shorter ICU and hospital length of stay.[50] Early mobility has been incorporated into the Pain, Agitation, and Delirium Clinical Practice Guidelines because of the positive impact on prevention of PICS.[51] Additionally, early mobility is an element of the ABCDE Bundle, which is a practical, multidisciplinary, evidence-based approach to preventing PICS in mechanically ventilated patients.[52] Mobilizing ICU patients is a challenge and many ICUs are not equipped with adequate physical therapy services or supportive equipment. Furthermore, for many hospitals this represents a culture change that requires evolved thinking and collaboration among nurses, physicians, and respiratory and physical therapists. Administrators must be convinced of the need for additional resources to facilitate mobilizing ICU patients, and nurses must translate the positive clinical

Box 1
Medical Research Council muscle strength scores

No movement or contraction = 0

Palpable contraction, no movement observed = 1

Movement at the joint with gravity eliminated = 2

Able to move the joint against gravity = 3

Able to move the joint against resistance, less than normal = 4

Fully normal strength = 5

Measure in three muscle groups bilaterally in upper and lower extremities; total normal score = 60.

From Medical Research Council. Aids to the examination of the peripheral nervous system. London: Her Majesty's Stationary Office; 1976.

outcomes to financial outcomes (ie, the costs of longer ventilator dependence and ICU stays) to make the argument. Fortunately, there is a sound research base on which to make a case for the clinical and economic advantages to early mobility.

SUMMARY

Sedation is a necessary aspect of managing critical illness. Control of agitation and anxiety to maximize the therapeutic management plan and promote healing are the overriding goals of sedation in the ICU. Oversedation negates many of the restorative processes, however, and contributes to multiple complications most of which are part of the PICS, including prolonged immobility and the deleterious consequences of disuse atrophy and deteriorating physical function; risk for cognitive impairment; and psychiatric symptoms, compromising quality of life for survivors of critical illness. Critically ill patients have multiple causes of persistent, severe weakness, as illustrated by the case example described at the beginning of this article. Oversedation acts synergistically with other risk factors and perpetuates a cycle of inactivity, muscle wasting, and extreme weakness, along with cognitive and psychiatric impairment. Oversedation increases ventilator days and prolongs ICU length of stay, which translates into exponential cost increases. Improved methods of evaluating appropriate levels of sedation, strategies in medication delivery and sedative selection, and nonburdensome feasible ways to assess muscle strength and integrity contribute to improved functional outcomes for patients following critical illness.

REFERENCES

1. Needham DM, Davidson J, Cohen H, et al. Improving long-term outcomes after discharge from intensive care unit: report from a stakeholders' conference. Crit Care Med 2012;40(2):502–9.
2. Mikkelsen ME, Iwashyna TJ, Thompson C. Why ICU clinicians need to care about post-intensive care syndrome. Critical Connections 2015;14(4):1, 9.
3. Desai SV, Law TJ, Needham DM. Long-term complications of critical care. Crit Care Med 2011;39(2):371–9.
4. Schelling G, Stoll C, Vogelmeier C, et al. Pulmonary function and health-related quality of life in a sample of long-term survivors of the acute respiratory distress syndrome. Intensive Care Med 2000;26(9):1304–11.
5. Hough CL, Steinberg KP, Taylor TB, et al. Intensive care unit-acquired neuromyopathy and corticosteroids in survivors of persistent ARDS. Intensive Care Med 2009;35(1):63–8.
6. Stevens RD, Dowdy DW, Michaels RK, et al. Neuromuscular dysfunction acquired in critical illness: a systematic review. Intensive Care Med 2007;33:1876–91.
7. de Jonghe B, Lacherade JC, Sharshar T, et al. Intensive care unit-acquired weakness: risk factors and prevention. Crit Care Med 2009;37(10 Suppl):S309–15.
8. Bolton CF, Gilbert JJ, Hahn AF, et al. Polyneuropathy in critically ill patients. J Neurol Neurosurg Psychiatry 1984;47:1223–31.
9. Latronico N, Peli E, Botteri M. Critical illness myopathy and neuropathy. Curr Opin Crit Care 2005;11(2):126–32.
10. Stevens RD, Marshall SA, Cornblath DR, et al. A framework for diagnosing and classifying intensive care unit-acquired weakness. Crit Care Med 2009;37(10 Suppl):S299–308.
11. Fletcher SN, Kennedy DD, Ghosh IR, et al. Persistent neuromuscular and neurophysiologic abnormalities in long-term survivors of prolonged critical illness. Crit Care Med 2003;31:1012–6.

12. De Jonghe B, Sharshar T, Lefaucheur JP, et al. Paresis acquired in the intensive care unit a prospective multicenter study. JAMA 2002;288(22):2859–67.
13. Ramsay DA, Zochdne DW, Robertson DM, et al. A syndrome of acute severe muscle necrosis in intensive care unit patients. J Neuropathol Exp Neurol 1993; 52(4):387–98.
14. Kasper CE, Talbot LA, Gaines JM. Skeletal muscle damage and recovery. AACN Clin Issues 2002;13(2):237–47.
15. Chambers MA, Moylan JS, Reid MB. Physical inactivity and muscle weakness in the critically ill. Crit Care Med 2009;37(10 Suppl):S337–46.
16. van der Schaaf M, Beelen A, Dongelmans DA, et al. Functional status after intensive care unit: a challenge for rehabilitation professionals to improve outcome. J Rehabil Med 2009;41(5):360–6.
17. Chaboyer W, Grace J. Following the path of ICU survivors: a quality improvement activity. Nurs Crit Care 2003;8(4):149–55.
18. Jackson JC, Pandharipande PP, Girard TD, et al. Depression, posttraumatic stress disorder, and functional disability in survivors of critical illness: results from the BRAIN ICU (Bringing to light the Risk Factors and Incidence of Neuropsychological dysfunction in ICU survivors) Investigation: a longitudinal cohort study. Lancet Respir Med 2014;2(5):369–79.
19. Beck AT, Steer RA, Brown G. BDI-II depression inventory manual. New York: Harcourt Brace; 1996.
20. Davydow DS, Gifford JM, Desai SV, et al. Depression in general intensive care unit survivors: a systematic review. Intensive Care Med 2009;35(5):796–809.
21. Davydow DS, Desai SV, Needham DM, et al. Psychiatric morbidity in survivors of acute respiratory distress syndrome: a systematic review. Psychosom Med 2008; 70:512–9.
22. Horowitz M, Wilner N, Alvarez W. Impact of event scale: a measure of subjective stress. Psychosom Med 1979;41:209–18.
23. Blanchard EB, Jones-Alexander J, Buckley TC, et al. Psychometric properties of the PTSD checklist. Behav Res Ther 1996;34:669–73.
24. Pandharipande P, Shintani A, Peterson J, et al. Lorezapam is an independent risk factor for transitioning to delirium in intensive care unit patients. Anesthesiology 2006;104:21–6.
25. Zaal IJ, Devlin JW, Hazelbag M, et al. Benzodiazepine-associated delirium in critically ill patients. Intensive Care Med 2015;41(12):2130–7.
26. Jackson JC, Girard TD, Gordon SM, et al. Long-term cognitive and psychological outcomes in the awakening and breathing controlled trial. Am J Respir Crit Care Med 2010;182:183–91.
27. Cuthbertson BH, Roughton S, Jenkinson D, et al. Quality of life in the five years after intensive care: a cohort study. Crit Care Med 2010;14(1):R6.
28. Bioc JJ, Magee C, Cucchi J, et al. Cost effectiveness of a benzodiazepine vs a nonbenzodiazepine-based sedation regimen for mechanically ventilated, critically ill adults. J Crit Care 2014;29(5):753–7.
29. Fraser GL, Devlin JW, Worby CP, et al. Benzodiazepine vs nonbenzodiazepine-based sedation for mechanically ventilated, critically ill adults: a systematic review and meta-analysis of randomized trials. Crit Care Med 2013;41(Suppl 9): S530–8.
30. Carrasco G. Instruments for monitoring intensive care unit sedation. Crit Care 2000;4(4):217–25.
31. Ramsay M, Savage T, Simpson BRJ, et al. Controlled sedation with alphaxalone/alphadalone. BMJ 1974;2:656–9.

32. Chernik DA, Gillings D, Laine H, et al. Validity and reliability of the Observer's Assessment of Alertness/Sedation scale: study with intravenous midazolam. J Clin Psychopharmacol 1990;10(4):244–51.
33. Harris CE, O'Donnell C, MacMillan RR. Use of propofol infusion for sedation of patients undergoing haemofiltration: assessment of the effect of haemofiltration on the level of sedation and on blood propofol concentration. J Drug Dev 1991;(Suppl 3):37–9.
34. Riker RR, Picard JT, Fraser GL. Prospective evaluation of the sedation agitation scale for adult critically ill patients. Crit Care Med 1999;27(7):1325–9.
35. Olleveant N, Humphris G, Roe B. A reliability study of the modified new Sheffield Sedation Scale. Nurs Crit Care 1998;3(2):83–8.
36. Devlin JW, Boleski G, Mylnarek M, et al. Motor activity assessment scale: a valid and reliable sedation scale for use with mechanically ventilated patients in an adult surgical intensive care unit. Crit Care Med 1999;27(7):1271–5.
37. de Lemos J, Tweeddale M, Chittock D. Measuring quality of sedation in adult mechanically ventilated critically ill patients. J Clin Epidemiol 2000;53:908–19.
38. Fraser GL, Riker R. Monitoring sedation, agitation, analgesia, and delirium in critically ill adult patients. Crit Care Clin 2001;17:1–21.
39. Sessler CN, Gosnell MS, Grap MJ, et al. The Richmond Agitation-Sedation Scale: validity and reliability in adult intensive care unit patients. Am J Respir Crit Care Med 2002;166:1338–44.
40. De Jonghe BD, Cook D, Griffith L, et al. Adaptation to the intensive care unit environment (ATICE): development and validation of a new sedation assessment instrument. Crit Care Med 2003;31(9):2344–54.
41. Weinert CR, McFarland L. The state of intubated ICU patient: development of a two-dimensional sedation rating scale for critically ill adults. Chest 2004;126:1883–90.
42. Binnekade JM, Vroom MB, de Vos R, et al. The reliability and validity of a new and simple method to measure sedation levels in intensive care patients: a pilot study. Heart Lung 2006;35(2):137–43.
43. Mirski MA, LeDroux SN, Lewin JJ, et al. Validity and reliability of an intuitive conscious sedation scoring tool: the nursing instrument for the communication of sedation. Crit Care Med 2010;38(8):1674–84.
44. Robinson BR, Berube M, Barr J, et al. Psychometric analysis of subjective sedation scales in critically ill adults. Crit Care Med 2013;41(9 Suppl 1):S16–29.
45. Kress JP, Pohlman AS, O'Connor MF, et al. Daily interruption of sedative infusions in critically ill patients undergoing mechanical ventilation. N Engl J Med 2000;342(20):1471–7.
46. Balas MC, Vaselevskis EE, Olsen KM, et al. Effectiveness and safety of the awakening and breathing coordination, delirium monitoring/management, and early exercise/mobility bundle. Crit Care Med 2014;42(5):1024–36.
47. Treggiari MM, Romand JA, Yanez D, et al. Randomized trial of light versus deep sedation on mental health after critical illness. Crit Care Med 2009;37(9):2527–34.
48. Medical Research Council. Aids to the examination of the peripheral nervous system. London: Her Majesty's Stationary Office; 1976.
49. Chlan LL, Tracy MF, Guttormson J, et al. Peripheral muscle strength and correlates of muscle weakness in patients receiving mechanical ventilation. Am J Crit Care 2015;24(6):e91–8.
50. Morris PE, Goad A, Thompson C, et al. Early intensive care unit mobility therapy in the treatment of acute respiratory failure. Crit Care Med 2008;36(8):1–8.

51. Barr J, Fraser GL, Puntillo K, et al. Implementation of the Pain, Agitation, and Delirium Clinical Practice Guidelines and promoting patient mobility to prevent post-intensive care syndrome. Crit Care Med 2013;41(9 Suppl):S136–40.
52. Morandi A, Brummel NE, Ely EW. Sedation, delirium and mechanical ventilation: the ABCDE approach. Curr Opin Crit Care 2011;17(1):43–9.

Application of Clinical Practice Guidelines for Pain, Agitation, and Delirium

Anna Krupp, MS, RN[a], Michele C. Balas, PhD, RN[b,*]

KEYWORDS

• Sedation • Pain • Agitation • Delirium • Intensive care unit • Guidelines

KEY POINTS

- Sedative medications are often administered to critically ill patients to prevent and manage commonly experienced and distressful symptoms.
- A recent clinical practice guideline released by the American College of Critical Care Medicine provides clinicians an integrated and evidence-based approach to managing pain, agitation, and delirium in the critically ill.
- Successful adoption of sedation guidelines requires clinicians to acknowledge the prevalence and patient-centered outcomes associated with pain, agitation, and delirium and the hazards of deep sedation.
- Strategies, such as using valid and reliable PAD assessment tools, setting desired sedation target levels, and choosing appropriate sedative medications, may improve patient outcomes.
- Sedative medication exposure may also be reduced through the use of nonpharmacologic symptom management strategies and enhanced interprofessional collaboration.

INTRODUCTION

Tim is a 50-year-old man who presented to the emergency department with shortness of breath; light headedness; chest pain; and a 2-day history of fever, muscle aches, and fatigue. Before his present illness, Tim was employed full-time as an interstate truck driver. He has a history of hypertension that is treated with oral medication,

---

Disclosure Statement: Ms A. Krupp has nothing to disclose. Dr M.C. Balas has received past honoraria for CME activities from: Dignity Health, the Society of Critical Care Medicine, the National Hartford Center for Gerontological Nursing Excellence/The John A. Hartford Foundation Institute for Geriatric Nursing/American Association of Colleges of Nursing, Hill-Rom, Hospira, and the France Foundation.

[a] Department of Nursing and Patient Care Services, University of Wisconsin Hospital and Clinics, 600 Highland Avenue, C7/305, Madison, WI 53792, USA; [b] Center of Excellence in Critical and Complex Care, College of Nursing, The Ohio State University, 368 Newton Hall, 1585 Neil Avenue, Columbus, OH 43210, USA
* Corresponding author.
E-mail address: balas.17@osu.edu

Crit Care Nurs Clin N Am 28 (2016) 241–252
http://dx.doi.org/10.1016/j.cnc.2016.02.001
ccnursing.theclinics.com
0899-5885/16/$ – see front matter

and otherwise he does not routinely seek medical care. Within 30 minutes of arrival to the emergency department, Tim was intubated for respiratory failure and admitted to the medical intensive care unit (ICU) with a diagnosis of pneumonia. On arrival to the ICU Tim is frowning, attempting to sit up, and touching his endotracheal tube. He has not received any medications since intubation 90 minutes ago. What evidence-based symptom management strategies should be prioritized to facilitate Tim's successful transition to the ICU?

Within the next 24 hours, Tim's respiratory failure has become progressively more severe and he is diagnosed with acute respiratory distress syndrome. His fraction of inspired oxygen has been increased from 0.6 to 0.8 in the past 4 hours, resulting in a slight increase in his Pa_{O_2} to 60 mm Hg. His target sedation level is drowsy; however, his actual sedation level is agitated with frequent nonpurposeful movement, and he has had increasing ventilator dyssynchrony. He has signs of pain and last delirium assessment was positive. Soft wrist restraints were initiated overnight after repeated movements toward his endotracheal tube. What symptom management interventions should be prioritized?

Despite improving ventilator dyssynchrony with treatment of pain and agitation with medications, Tim's Pa_{O_2} remains critically low. Venovenous extracorporeal membrane oxygenation (ECMO) is initiated via femoral cannulation. Over the course of the next 4 days Tim remains on bedrest. Four days after initiating ECMO Tim's oxygenation improves. ECMO is weaned off and his fraction of inspired oxygen requirement is 0.5. His target score is alert and calm, yet his actual sedation score is light sedation. His pain score is negative and delirium assessment remains positive. He has received two doses of intravenous analgesic medication and two doses of intravenous benzodiazepine medication over the past 24 hours in response to pain and anxiety symptoms. How will ventilator discontinuation be coordinated? What additional interventions should be implemented for resolving Tim's delirium? What is his goal for early mobility?

At each stage of Tim's course in the ICU, questions about pain, agitation, sedation, delirium, and associated clinical outcomes surfaced. These questions are not uncommon for any adult patient receiving mechanical ventilation in the ICU setting and answers to these clinical questions require an evidence-based approach.

CLINICAL PRACTICE GUIDELINES FOR THE MANAGEMENT OF PAIN, AGITATION, AND DELIRIUM IN ADULT PATIENTS IN THE INTENSIVE CARE UNIT

Critically ill patients, such as Tim, experience several severe, distressing, and often life-altering symptoms during their ICU stay.[1] Strong evidence generated over the last few decades suggests the way these symptoms are assessed and managed in the ICU setting is strongly linked to a patient's ability to recover from a serious or life-threatening illness or injury.[2] In 2013, the American College of Critical Care Medicine published its Clinical Practice Guidelines for the Management of Pain, Agitation, and Delirium in Adult Patients in the ICU.[2] The goal of the guideline is to recommend best practices for managing pain, agitation, and delirium (PAD) to improve patient-centered outcomes in critically ill adults. Since its dissemination, numerous hospitals throughout the world are updating their PAD-related policies and procedures, educating clinicians regarding the guideline's major suggestions and recommendations, and engaging critically ill patients and their families to become more actively involved in their ICU care.[3] This article illustrates how the new PAD guidelines could be applied in everyday clinical practice.

ACKNOWLEDGE THE INCIDENCE AND OUTCOMES OF PAIN, AGITATION, AND DELIRIUM IN THE INTENSIVE CARE UNIT

A large portion of the latest PAD guidelines is devoted to succinctly summarizing the incidence and outcomes of pain, agitation, oversedation, and delirium in the ICU. This is an important initial teaching point for those involved with active guideline implementation efforts because many ICU providers may not fully appreciate the magnitude of the problem. For example, pain, occurring in more than 70% of medical, surgical, and cardiothoracic ICU patients,[4,5] is by far one of the most prevalent, distressing, and undertreated physical symptoms experienced by critically ill patients.[2] The pain experienced by persons requiring mechanical ventilation occurs at rest and with routine ICU activities, such as wound care, drain removal, tracheal suctioning, and turning.[6] Agitation and anxiety, common symptoms in mechanically ventilated ICU patients,[2] may not only lead to the accidental self-removal of endotracheal and other critical tubes and lines,[7] but also cause an increase in circulating catecholamines and an increased stress response potentially worsening myocardial ischemia, wound healing, and immune responses.[8] Delirium, a syndrome affecting up to two-thirds of mechanically ventilated ICU patients,[9,10] is a strong, independent predictor of short- and long-term mortality, longer ICU and hospital length of stay, and prolonged mechanical ventilation.

The guidelines also emphasize that the negative physical, mental, and cognitive health consequences of developing PAD in the ICU setting are important and frequently long-lasting.[2] For example, the PAD guideline acknowledges ICU pain is associated with insufficient sleep,[11] traumatic memories,[12] posttraumatic stress disorder,[13,14] chronic pain,[2] and lower health-related quality of life.[14] Delirium is an important independent predictor of substantial functional decline, new institutionalization, and neurocognitive deficits so severe that they are similar to those seen in persons suffering from moderate traumatic brain injury or mild Alzheimer disease.[10,15–19] **Fig. 1** illustrates patient consequences of fragmented ICU care and the importance of an integrated approach to assess and manage ICU symptoms. Given the frequency and outcomes associated with commonly experienced ICU symptoms, the guidelines

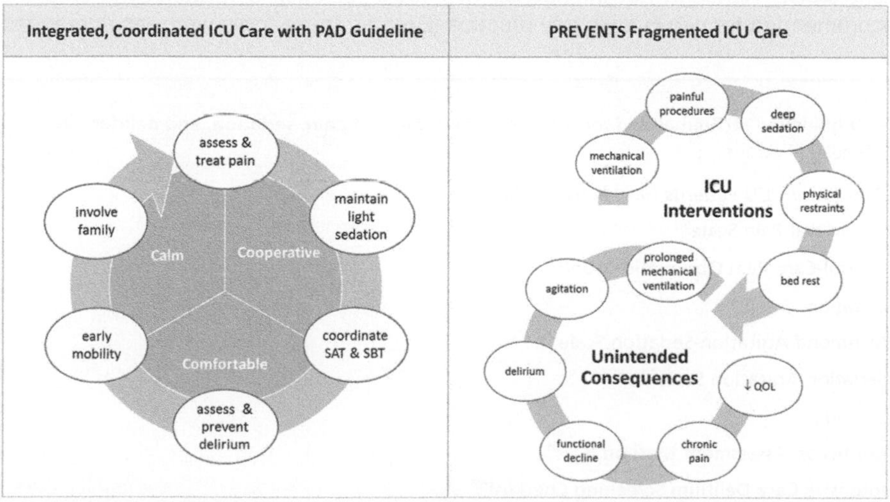

Fig. 1. Benefits of comprehensive PAD guideline. QOL, quality of life; SAT, spontaneous awakening trial; SBT, spontaneous breathing trial.

suggest it is essential providers implement integrated, evidence-based, and patient-centered symptom management protocols into their everyday practice.[2] This process, importantly, should begin at the time of ICU admission.

RECOGNIZE MANY FACTORS COMPLICATE EFFECTIVE PAIN, AGITATION, AND DELIRIUM ASSESSMENT, PREVENTION, AND MANAGEMENT

The guidelines acknowledge that several factors complicate ICU providers' ability to effectively assess, prevent, and manage PAD in critically ill patients. Ideally, symptoms are reported and rated by patients themselves.[20] This is challenging in mechanically ventilated patients who are often unable to self-report their symptoms either verbally or nonverbally because of underlying disease processes (eg, primary neurologic injury), the use of tubes that impede normal speech (eg, endotracheal tubes, tracheostomies), treatments that make communication impossible (eg, administration of neuromuscular blockade agents), or the application of physical restraints that limit the use of hand gestures or written communication.[21,22] Another complicating factor is mechanically ventilated patients are frequently exposed to particularly high-risk medication classes (eg, opioids, sedatives, hypnotics, antipsychotics) during their ICU stay.[2] Although these medications are often given to treat a patient's symptoms, as outlined in the PAD guideline[2] their administration may be associated with substantial harm. For example, these medications often complicate effective symptom assessment by further reducing a patient's level of consciousness and hence their ability to self-report, paradoxically increase the risk for other syndromes (eg, benzodiazepines administered for agitation are known to increase the risk for delirium), and heighten the risk of iatrogenic injury caused by the effects of deep sedation (eg, prolonged mechanical ventilation and elevated mortality).[2,23–26]

BEGIN WITH ROUTINE PAIN, AGITATION, AND DELIRIUM MONITORING USING VALID AND RELIABLE TOOLS

Given these challenges, the PAD guideline emphasizes the importance of routine pain, agitation/sedation, and delirium monitoring using valid and reliable behavioral assessment tools.[2] Although not intentional, two tools for each symptom/syndrome are recommended for use in everyday practice (**Box 1**). These tools were recommended

Box 1
PAD guideline recommended tools for the assessment of pain, sedation, and delirium in critically ill adults

Pain (Adult ICU Patients Unable to Self-Report)

Behavioral Pain Scale[56]

Critical-Care Pain Observation Tool[57]

Sedation

Richmond Agitation-Sedation Scale[33]

Sedation-Agitation Scale[34]

Delirium

Confusion Assessment Method ICU[58]

Intensive Care Delirium Screening Checklist[59]

Data from Refs.[33,34,56–59]

for their strong psychometric properties. Although the guideline does not clearly define the term "routine," the PAD care bundle provided in the document suggests assessing pain and agitation four or more times per shift and when necessary and delirium each shift and when necessary.[2] Several research and quality improvement projects to date have shown implementing these assessment tools into everyday care is feasible[27–29] and, when bundled with other evidence-based interventions, leads to improved patient outcomes.[30]

Several points regarding pain assessment in the critically ill warrant further discussion. First, it is important to recognize that a patient's "self-report" remains the gold standard of pain assessment.[20] Given that their level of consciousness is not too impaired because of their severity of illness or receipt of sedative medications, many mechanically ventilated and nonmechanically ventilated patients are able to express pain presence and intensity during their ICU stay. According to research by Chanques and coworkers,[31] a 0 to 10 Numeric Rating Scale is the most valid, reliable, and feasible method of pain self-report in the critically ill. In patients able to communicate, either verbally or nonverbally, several other methods could be used to empower them to be able to self-report their pain including using multisymptom assessment tools, short symptom word lists, body outline diagrams, and simply asking patients to point to the places where they are feeling pain.[20] Given the emphasis placed in the PAD guidelines on maintaining light levels of sedation, described in greater detail next, it is likely that these pain self-report measures will be used more frequently in the ICU setting.

It is equally important for clinicians to recognize that in some critically ill patients it may not be possible to use either a patient's self-report or the PAD guideline recommended behavioral pain scales to fully understand the patient's pain experience. In the literature, two other approaches have been recommended to facilitate pain assessment in these types of patients. These two approaches include using a patient's family members for proxy pain assessment and presuming pain is present in situations in which communicative patients typically report such distress.[20] The role objective measures of brain function play in sedation monitoring in the ICU is discussed more fully in this issue (see Olson DM, Phillips K, Graffagnino C: Towards Solving the Sedation-Assessment Conundrum: Neurofunction Monitoring).

MAINTAIN CRITICALLY ILL PATIENTS IN A LIGHT, RATHER THAN DEEP, LEVEL OF SEDATION

Unless clinically contraindicated, the guidelines recommend that sedative medications be titrated to maintain a light, rather than deep, level of sedation in adult ICU patients.[32] Although the examples of light and deep sedation levels are broadly defined in the guideline itself (ie, ranging from a patient who is arousable and able to purposefully follow simple commands to a patient who is unarousable to painful stimuli), in the accompanying PAD care bundle more specific examples are given. For example, light sedation in the bundle is defined as a Richmond Agitation Sedation Score[33] of -1 to -2 and a Sedation-Agitation Scale[34] of 3; whereas deep sedation is defined as a Richmond Agitation Sedation Score of -3 to -5 and a Sedation-Agitation Scale of 1 to 2. The more concrete definitions (given they come with objective sedation/agitation assessment scores) may be more helpful to clinicians trying to implement this important recommendation into everyday practice.

Two strategies are recommended in the PAD guideline to achieve light levels of sedation in the critically ill. These strategies include the use of daily sedation interruption (also known as spontaneous awakening trials) or using protocols to maintain light sedation. Although not always explicitly defined, inherent to both strategies is the use of sedation "target" levels. A target sedation level, used primarily to facilitate ICU team communication and common goal setting,[35] is a set, objective measure of the desired level of sedation needed to maintain patient comfort and facilitate needed ICU interventions. Ideally, the target sedation score should be set by the ICU team on daily interprofessional rounds, be based on the individual patient's need, formulated considering goals of care, and aimed achieving the highest level of arousal that is safely possible for the patient. Using a target sedation score then helps providers make the critical decisions needed when using either of the recommended strategies for achieving light levels of sedation (ie, daily sedation interruption or protocolized sedation) recommended in the PAD guideline.

CHOOSE THE RIGHT MEDICATION FOR THE SYMPTOM/SYNDROME TO BE PREVENTED OR MANAGED

The PAD guideline emphasizes the importance of choosing the "right" sedative medication for the "right" reason. For example, the guidelines suggest using an analgesia-first sedation strategy in mechanically ventilated patients. An analgesia-first approach, a strategy that focuses on treating pain before using other sedative medications, may not only obliterate the need for administration of other sedative medications all together but lead to improved patient outcomes.[36] Although intravenous opioids are recommended as the first-line drug choice to treat nonneuropathic pain in critically ill adults,[2] the guidelines also suggest providers consider using nonopioid analgesics to decrease the amount of opioids administered and decrease the risk of opioid-related side effects. Other strategies that may reduce pain incidence and severity in the critically ill include using preemptive analgesia and/or nonpharmacologic interventions, enterally administered gabapentin or carbamazepine for the treatment of neuropathic pain, and thoracic epidural anesthesia/analgesia for patients undergoing abdominal aortic aneurysms and/or rib fractures.[2]

In those circumstances where a patient's pain is adequately controlled, yet the patient is not at their ideal sedation target, clinicians then need to explore other sedation options weighing each's potential risk and benefits. The guidelines suggest strategies using nonbenzodiazepine (ie, either propofol or dexmedetomidine) sedatives may be preferred over sedation with benzodiazepines,[2] because the latter (ie, benzodiazepines) may increase ICU length of stay,[37] the duration of mechanical ventilation,[37] and the occurrence of delirium.[23]

APPLY NONPHARMACOLOGIC PAIN, AGITATION, AND DELIRIUM PREVENTION AND MANAGEMENT INTERVENTIONS

Although many treatment recommendations in the guidelines include the use of medications, early mobility and sleep promotion are two nonpharmacologic interventions recommended to reduce the occurrence and length of delirium.[2] Early mobility has been established as a safe and feasible intervention to improve functional outcomes and duration of delirium.[38] Early mobility interventions are typically delivered using a team approach that may include rehabilitation therapists, nurses, respiratory therapists, and/or aides. Several early mobility protocols have been published to describe the step-wise process of advancing activity from in-bed exercises to dangling, standing, and walking.[39–41] The purpose of a mobility protocol is to describe clear criteria to advance a patient's physical activity to their prehospital abilities as soon as a patient meets defined physiologic criteria. Mobility protocols also identify safety parameters, such as respiratory, cardiovascular, and neurologic characteristics for participation in early mobility. Because of its known benefits, early mobility programs are beginning to include sicker and sicker patients. For example, some centers now have early mobility protocols that would include such patients as Tim even when he was undergoing ECMO therapy.[42,43]

Multiple patient, personnel, and organizational barriers to early mobility programs have unfortunately been identified.[44,45] Implementation of the PAD guidelines is one solution to overcoming one of the more common patient barriers: oversedation. One of the requirements for a successful early mobility program is that pain and sedation treatment are at targeted goals before advancing activity. Clearly, the more deeply sedated a patient is the less likely they are to be able to participate in physical activity. Implementation of the PAD guidelines helps break the vicious cycle of deep sedation, immobility, and prolonged mechanical ventilation by its emphasis on using strategies (ie, daily sedation interruption and protocolized sedation) aimed at maintaining patients in a more cognitively and physically engaged state.

Developing day/night routines is another nonpharmacologic intervention to promote sleep and reduce the development of delirium.[46] Sleep deprivation is a modifiable risk factor for the development of delirium and the guidelines recommend environmental and structural interventions to organize times awake and protected sleep time.[2] Interventions to promote day and night routines include arranging light and stimuli to mimic a nonhospital schedule, such as light and activity during daylight, uninterrupted periods of time during the night, scheduled rest time, and clustering activities. The quality of sleep is also closely related to pain and sedation management, because undertreatment of pain may disrupt sleep and overtreatment of sedation may appear to be restful, but instead decreases the amount of deeper sleep stages.[46] Therefore, the PAD recommendations for treatment of pain and sedation, in addition to nonpharmacologic interventions, are important for sleep promotion.

IMPORTANCE OF INTERPROFESSIONAL COLLABORATION WHEN IMPLEMENTING THE PAIN, AGITATION, AND DELIRIUM GUIDELINE

The PAD guidelines contain process recommendations in addition to the clinical recommendations previously discussed. These process recommendations include using an interprofessional team to develop and implement tools, such as protocols, order sets, and rounding checklists.[2] The use of a bundled protocol to implement recommendations for coordinating goal-directed sedation with spontaneous breathing trials, delirium prevention, and early mobility has been effective in improving patient outcomes.[30,47] For example, the ABCDEF bundle (*A*ssess, prevent, and manage pain; *B*oth spontaneous awakening trials and spontaneous breathing trials; *C*hoice of analgesia and sedation; assess, prevent, and manage *D*elirium; *E*arly mobility and exercise; and *F*amily engagement and empowerment) includes many of the PAD guideline recommendations that are operationalized in a clearly defined manner but is flexible enough to enable institutions to tweak the interventions to meet the unique needs of its patients and its own culture.[3] Critically ill patients managed with the original ABCDEF bundle spent 3 more days breathing without assistance, experienced less delirium, and were more likely to be mobilized during their ICU stay than patients treated with usual care.[30]

Protocols are a tool to implement guideline recommendations at the point of care. Yet overall, protocols do not always consistently impact patient outcomes.[48] Having an existing culture of patient safety and resources to support protocol implementation, such as planning and training, are factors that influence the success of consistent protocol use in daily practice.[49] The PAD guidelines recognize the importance of local culture in establishing successful practice change, and therefore, do not prescribe specific implementation requirements, but instead acknowledge implementation factors to consider at a unit or organizational level.

Another noteworthy component of the PAD guideline is a focus on the interprofessional team. Successful teams identify and include all roles in all phases of practice change: development, implementation, and sustainment.[50] PAD guideline recommendations impact virtually all disciplines that provide care in the ICU, and therefore interprofessional involvement is critical. In addition to advanced practice nurses, physicians, and physician assistants, specific roles identified for successful implementation of components of the PAD guidelines include pharmacists,[51] respiratory therapists,[52] rehabilitation therapists,[53] and nurses.[35,54] Equally, it is critical to recognize that PAD recommendations are interdependent on one another and therefore ICU practitioners need to be aware of the sum and parts of the PAD guidelines.[55] One method for communicating and coordinating patient-specific assessment and management of PAD is daily interprofessional rounds. Nurses have important contextual patient assessment, intervention, and response data for all elements of the PAD recommendations and are responsible for patient care coordination. A "brain road map" is one example of a tool to focus nurse presentation of PAD content, and includes (1) target sedation score, (2) current sedation and delirium score, and (3) interventions.[35] Having structures in place, such as protocols and interdisciplinary communication, is necessary for supporting the complex coordination of these interdependent practice recommendations.

CAPITALIZING ON AVAILABLE RESOURCES

Since publication of the PAD guidelines in 2013 multiple publications and resources have been disseminated to support PAD practice changes. The American Association of Critical Care Nurses (http://www.aacn.org) and the Society for Critical Care Medicine (http://www.iculiberation.org) have organized toolkits with online access to education and implementation materials. Another powerful resource available online is a collection of videos from patients and family members with ICU experiences that reinforce the benefits of PAD prevention (http://www.icudelirium.org). These resources are available as examples of how processes can be customized and standardized at the unit or organizational level to improve the success of the PAD recommendations being translated into practice change.

SUMMARY

Critically ill patients experience several severe and distressing symptoms during their ICU stay that often have long-term consequences. The PAD guideline provides best practices for the assessment, management, and prevention of PAD, which in turn improves the care and outcomes for ICU patients. A summary of strategies to implement this guideline into daily practice includes using valid and reliable PAD assessment tools; setting a desired sedation level target and focusing on light sedation; choosing appropriate sedative medications; using nonpharmacologic symptom management strategies; and engaging patients, significant others, and all members of the interprofessional team to actively partner in delivering care. The combined effect of the PAD recommendations provides the foundation for a standard of care for ICU patients and the opportunity to improve care and long-term outcomes for critically ill patients.

REFERENCES

1. Puntillo KA, Arai S, Cohen NH, et al. Symptoms experienced by intensive care unit patients at high risk of dying. Crit Care Med 2010;38(11):2155–60.
2. Barr J, Fraser GL, Puntillo K, et al. Clinical practice guidelines for the management of pain, agitation, and delirium in adult patients in the intensive care unit. Crit Care Med 2013;41(1):263–306.
3. Balas M, Barnes-Daly M, Byrum D, et al. Helping critically ill patients and families thrive through an ABCDEF approach. Crit Connections 2015;14:1, 10.
4. Puntillo KA. Pain experiences of intensive care unit patients. Heart Lung 1990; 19(5 Pt 1):526–33.
5. Gélinas C. Management of pain in cardiac surgery ICU patients: have we improved over time? Intensive Crit Care Nurs 2007;23(5):298–303.
6. Puntillo KA, White C, Morris AB, et al. Patients' perceptions and responses to procedural pain: results from Thunder Project II. Am J Crit Care 2001;10(4): 238–51, 214.
7. Sessler CN, Riker RR, Ramsay MA. Evaluating and monitoring sedation, arousal, and agitation in the ICU. Semin Respir Crit Care Med 2013;34(2):169–78.
8. Vileikyte L. Stress and wound healing. Clin Dermatol 2007;25(1):49–55.
9. Milbrandt EB, Deppen S, Harrison PL, et al. Costs associated with delirium in mechanically ventilated patients. Crit Care Med 2004;32(4):955–62.
10. Ely EW, Shintani A, Truman B, et al. Delirium as a predictor of mortality in mechanically ventilated patients in the intensive care unit. JAMA 2004;291(14):1753–62.
11. Jones J, Hoggart B, Withey J, et al. What the patients say: a study of reactions to an intensive care unit. Intensive Care Med 1979;5(2):89–92.
12. Gustav S, Markus R, Benno R, et al. Exposure to high stress in the intensive care unit may have negative effects on health-related quality-of-life outcomes after cardiac surgery. Crit Care Med 2003;31(7):1971–80.
13. Granja C, Gomes E, Amaro A, et al. Understanding posttraumatic stress disorder-related symptoms after critical care: the early illness amnesia hypothesis. Crit Care Med 2008;36(10):2801–9.
14. Schelling G, Stoll C, Haller M, et al. Health-related quality of life and posttraumatic stress disorder in survivors of the acute respiratory distress syndrome. Crit Care Med 1998;26(4):651–9.
15. Shehabi Y, Riker RR, Bokesch PM, et al. Delirium duration and mortality in lightly sedated, mechanically ventilated intensive care patients. Crit Care Med 2010; 38(12):2311–8.
16. Pisani MA, Kong SY, Kasl SV, et al. Days of delirium are associated with 1-year mortality in an older intensive care unit population. Am J Respir Crit Care Med 2009;180(11):1092–7.
17. Girard TD, Jackson JC, Pandharipande PP, et al. Delirium as a predictor of long-term cognitive impairment in survivors of critical illness. Crit Care Med 2010; 38(7):1513–20.
18. Balas MC, Happ MB, Yang W, et al. Outcomes associated with delirium in older patients in surgical ICUs. Chest 2009;135(1):18–25.
19. Pandharipande PP, Girard TD, Jackson JC, et al. Long-term cognitive impairment after critical illness. N Engl J Med 2013;369(14):1306–16.
20. Puntillo K, Nelson J, Weissman D, et al. Palliative care in the ICU: relief of pain, dyspnea, and thirst-A report from the IPAL-ICU Advisory Board. Intensive Care Med 2014;40(2):235–48.

21. Tate JA, Sereika S, Divirgilio D, et al. Symptom communication during critical illness: the impact of age, delirium, and delirium presentation. J Gerontol Nurs 2013;39(8):28–38.
22. Happ MB, Garrett KL, Tate JA, et al. Effect of a multi-level intervention on nurse-patient communication in the intensive care unit: results of the SPEACS trial. Heart Lung 2014;43(2):89–98.
23. Pandharipande P, Shintani A, Peterson J, et al. Lorazepam is an independent risk factor for transitioning to delirium in intensive care unit patients. Anesthesiology 2006;104(1):21–6.
24. Pisani MA, Murphy TE, Araujo KL, et al. Benzodiazepine and opioid use and the duration of intensive care unit delirium in an older population. Crit Care Med 2009;37(1):177–83.
25. Mehta S, Cook D, Devlin JW, et al. Prevalence, risk factors, and outcomes of delirium in mechanically ventilated adults. Crit Care Med 2015;43(3):557–66, 510.
26. Shehabi Y, Bellomo R, Reade MC, et al. Early intensive care sedation predicts long-term mortality in ventilated critically ill patients. Am J Respir Crit Care Med 2012;186(8):724–31.
27. Pun BT, Gordon SM, Peterson JF, et al. Large-scale implementation of sedation and delirium monitoring in the intensive care unit: a report from two medical centers. Crit Care Med 2005;33(6):1199–205.
28. Vasilevskis EE, Morandi A, Boehm L, et al. Delirium and sedation recognition using validated instruments: reliability of bedside intensive care unit nursing assessments from 2007 to 2010. J Am Geriatr Soc 2011;59(Suppl 2):S249–55.
29. Devlin JW, Marquis F, Riker RR, et al. Combined didactic and scenario-based education improves the ability of intensive care unit staff to recognize delirium at the bedside. Crit Care 2008;12(1):R19.
30. Balas MC, Vasilevskis EE, Olsen KM, et al. Effectiveness and safety of the awakening and breathing coordination, delirium monitoring/management, and early exercise/mobility bundle. Crit Care Med 2014;42(5):1024–36.
31. Chanques G, Viel E, Constantin J-M, et al. The measurement of pain in intensive care unit: comparison of 5 self-report intensity scales. Pain 2010;151(3):711–21.
32. Herridge MS, Cheung AM, Tansey CM, et al. One-year outcomes in survivors of the acute respiratory distress syndrome. N Engl J Med 2003;348(8):683–93.
33. Sessler CN, Gosnell MS, Grap MJ, et al. The Richmond Agitation-Sedation Scale: validity and reliability in adult intensive care unit patients. Am J Respir Crit Care Med 2002;166(10):1338–44.
34. Riker RR, Picard JT, Fraser GL. Prospective evaluation of the Sedation-Agitation Scale for adult critically ill patients. Crit Care Med 1999;27(7):1325–9.
35. Balas MC, Vasilevskis EE, Burke WJ, et al. Critical care nurses' role in implementing the "ABCDE bundle" into practice. Crit Care Nurse 2012;32(2):35–8, 40–7; [quiz: 48].
36. Strøm T, Mortinussen T, Toft P. A protocol of no sedation for critically ill patients receiving mechanical ventilation: a randomised trial. Lancet 2010;375(9713):475–80.
37. Fraser GL, Devlin JW, Worby CP, et al. Benzodiazepine versus nonbenzodiazepine-based sedation for mechanically ventilated, critically Ill adults: a systematic review and meta-analysis of randomized trials. Crit Care Med 2013;41(9):S30–8.
38. Schweickert WD, Pohlman MC, Pohlman AS, et al. Early physical and occupational therapy in mechanically ventilated, critically ill patients: a randomised controlled trial. Lancet 2009;373(9678):1874–82.

39. Engel HJ, Needham DM, Morris PE, et al. ICU early mobilization: from recommendation to implementation at three medical. Crit Care Med 2013;41(9 Suppl 1): S69–80.
40. Timmerman RA. A mobility protocol for critically ill adults. Dimens Crit Care Nurs 2007;26(5):175.
41. Gosselink R, Bott J, Johnson M, et al. Physiotherapy for adult patients with critical illness: recommendations of the European Respiratory Society and European Society of Intensive Care Medicine task force on physiotherapy for critically ill patients. Intensive Care Med 2008;34(7):1188–99.
42. Hodgson C, Bellomo R, Berney S, et al. Early mobilization and recovery in mechanically ventilated patients in the ICU: a bi-national, multi-centre, prospective cohort study. Crit Care 2015;19:81.
43. Rahimi RA, Skrzat J, Reddy DR, et al. Physical rehabilitation of patients in the intensive care unit requiring extracorporeal membrane oxygenation: a small case series. Phys Ther 2013;93(2):248–55.
44. Leditschke A, Green M, Irvine J, et al. What are the barriers to mobilizing intensive care patients? Cardiopulm Phys Ther J 2012;23(1):26–9.
45. Jolley SE, Regan-Baggs J, Dickson RP, et al. Medical intensive care unit clinician attitudes and perceived barriers towards early mobilization of critically ill patients: a cross-sectional survey study. BMC Anesthesiol 2014;14:84.
46. Weinhouse GL, Schwab RJ, Watson PL, et al. Bench-to-bedside review: delirium in ICU patients - importance of sleep deprivation. Crit Care 2009;13(6):234.
47. Kram SL, DiBartolo MC, Hinderer K, et al. Implementation of the ABCDE bundle to improve patient outcomes in the intensive care unit in a rural community hospital. Dimens Crit Care Nurs 2015;34(5):250–8, 259.
48. Sevransky JE, Checkley W, Herrera P, et al. Protocols and hospital mortality in critically ill patients: the United States critical illness and injury trials group critical illness outcomes study. Crit Care Med 2015;43(10):2076–84.
49. Carrothers KM, Barr J, Spurlock B, et al. Contextual issues influencing implementation and outcomes associated with an integrated approach to managing pain, agitation, and delirium in adult ICUs. Crit Care Med 2013;41(9 Suppl 1):S128–35.
50. Gershengorn HB, Kocher R, Factor P. Management strategies to effect change in intensive care units: lessons from the world of business. Part III. Effectively effecting and sustaining change. Ann Am Thorac Soc 2014;11(3):454–7.
51. Preslaski CR, Lat I, MacLaren R, et al. Pharmacist contributions as members of the multidisciplinary ICU team. Chest 2013;144(5):1687–95.
52. Ely EW, Baker AM, Dunagan DP, et al. Effect on the duration of mechanical ventilation of identifying patients capable of breathing spontaneously. N Engl J Med 1996;335(25):1864–9.
53. Kayambu G, Boots R, Paratz J. Physical therapy for the critically ill in the ICU: a systematic review and meta-analysis. Crit Care Med 2013;41(6):1543–54.
54. Mansouri P, Javadpour S, Zand F, et al. Implementation of a protocol for integrated management of pain, agitation, and delirium can improve clinical outcomes in the intensive care unit: a randomized clinical trial. J Crit Care 2013; 28(6):918–22.
55. Barr J, Pandharipande PP. The pain, agitation, and delirium care bundle: synergistic benefits of implementing the 2013 Pain, Agitation, and Delirium Guidelines in an integrated and interdisciplinary fashion. Crit Care Med 2013;41(9 Suppl 1): S99–115.
56. Payen J, Bru O, Bosson J, et al. Assessing pain in critically ill sedated patients by using a behavioral pain scale. Crit Care Med 2001;29(12):2258–63.

57. Gélinas C, Fillion L, Puntillo KA, et al. Validation of the critical-care pain observation tool in adult patients. Am J Crit Care 2006;15(4):420–7.
58. Ely EW, Inouye SK, Bernard GR, et al. Delirium in mechanically ventilated patients: validity and reliability of the confusion assessment method for the intensive care unit (CAM-ICU). JAMA 2001;286(21):2703–10.
59. Bergeron N, Dubois MJ, Dumont M, et al. Intensive care delirium screening checklist: evaluation of a new screening tool. Intensive Care Med 2001;27(5):859–64.

Sleep Disturbances in Acutely Ill Patients with Cancer

Ellyn E. Matthews, PhD, RN, AOCNS, CBSM*, J. Mark Tanner, DNP, RN,
Natalie A. Dumont, BS

KEYWORDS

• Sleep • Cancer • Critical illness • Sleep deprivation • Intensive care • Sleep quality • Insomnia • Sleep disorders

KEY POINTS

- Intensive care units (ICUs) provide specialized care to patients at risk for serious complications of cancer or its treatment.
- ICU-related sleep disturbances in conjunction with cancer-related sleep disturbance risk factors pose a significant clinical problem for patients with cancer.
- Routine assessment of sleep disturbances using a variety of tools can provide the basis for new approaches to treatment of sleep during acute illness.
- Effective treatment of sleep disturbances includes managing cancer-related symptoms, and implementing pharmacologic, nonpharmacologic, and environmental interventions.
- Nurses are well positioned to promote sleep health and generate knowledge about sleep disturbance through research.

Sleep, a vital component of human life, provides necessary restorative, protective, and energy-conserving functions. Sleep disturbances and fatigue are the most common symptoms in adults with cancer.[1] New-onset sleep disturbance or deterioration of sleep quality and quantity is a pervasive and disabling problem linked to cancer surgery, chemotherapy, hematopoietic stem cell transplant (HCT), radiation therapy,[2–5] and cancer itself. Difficulty falling asleep (onset insomnia), maintaining sleep, and excessive daytime sleepiness that develop during acute cancer treatment can

Disclosure: The authors received no financial support for this article.
Conflicts of Interest: The authors declare no conflicts of interest with respect to the authorship and/or publication of this article. No work resembling the enclosed article has been published or is being submitted for publication elsewhere. All authors have read the final version of the article and have made a substantial contribution to the final article. The authors report no financial relationships with commercial interests.
Department of Nursing Science, College of Nursing, University of Arkansas for Medical Sciences, 4301 West Markham Street, #529, Little Rock, AR 72205, USA
* Corresponding author.
E-mail addresses: eematthews@uams.edu; ellyn.matthews@va.gov

Crit Care Nurs Clin N Am 28 (2016) 253–268
http://dx.doi.org/10.1016/j.cnc.2016.02.006 **ccnursing.theclinics.com**
0899-5885/16/$ – see front matter

become enduring concerns, persisting long after completion of cancer treatments.[6] Moreover, when patients with cancer develop critical conditions requiring intensive care unit (ICU) admission, sleep is further compromised.

Many patients in medical ICUs have preexisting sleep disorders, particularly older adults,[7] and others show new sleep disturbances and deprivation.[8–10] **Table 1** describes common sleep disorders that may be present in acutely ill patients with cancer. Impaired sleep is linked to increased mortality, slowed recovery, altered immune function, and impaired cognition.[11–13] ICUs provide specialized care to individuals at risk for acute life-threatening complications of cancer or its treatment, particularly those with hematologic cancers (eg, leukemia, lymphoma) and lung cancer.[14] Pulmonary complications requiring ventilation, dialysis for renal failure, sepsis, neurologic disorders, and cardiovascular problems requiring vasopressor support are the most common critical complications of cancer leading to ICU admission.[15,16] Patients undergoing HCT often are transferred to ICUs for acute graft-versus-host disease, alveolar hemorrhage, and veno-occlusive disease of the liver; and nearly one-third require mechanical ventilation.[15,17] Cancer treatment complications and monitoring negatively affect sleep in ICUs. Combined with vulnerability to sleep issues that arise from cancer, ICU-related sleep disturbances pose a significant clinical problem.

Despite the high prevalence of sleep disturbances, research suggests that the communication about sleep in patients with cancer is suboptimal[18] and sleep problems are not regularly assessed or adequately treated throughout the cancer trajectory.[19] However, many sleep problems and fatigue can be managed effectively. Recognition of the frequency and characteristics of cancer-related sleep disturbances can provide the basis of new approaches to supportive care during and after acute illness. This article, therefore, synthesizes current literature about the prevalence, causes, and factors contributing to sleep disturbance in the context of acute cancer care, describes the consequences of poor sleep, and presents appropriate assessment and treatment options.

PREVALENCE OF CANCER-RELATED SLEEP DISTURBANCE

The prevalence and severity of sleep disturbances in oncology populations is difficult to determine because of patient underreporting, inconsistent evaluation by health care providers, and disparate sleep measures. Estimates suggest that more than one-half of patients with cancer experience some degree of sleep disturbance.[20,21] In comparison, sleep disturbance affects only 10% to 15% of the general population.[22] Of note, cancer-related fatigue (CRF) is highly correlated with poor sleep and is estimated to occur in 50% to 90% of patients with cancer.[23]

Sleep disturbances worsen during hospitalization and intensive treatment when the need for restorative sleep is greatest.[24] For example, insomnia was the most distressing symptom reported by 32% of HCT patients (N = 76) on the day of transplant.[25] In another study, of patients undergoing HCT (N = 44), 32% reported sleep disturbance before hospital admission, 77% during the hospital stay, and 28% after discharge.[26] These participants averaged 337 minutes of total sleep with 36% reporting 300 minutes or less per night.[26] Similarly, Hacker and colleagues[5] reported a mean of only 232 minutes of total sleep as measured by actigraphy in patients during HCT (N = 40). Taken together, these studies suggest that sleep disturbance and deprivation is not a trivial health issue for patients with cancer during hospitalization and during acute phases of the cancer trajectory.

CAUSES AND RISK FACTORS

Risk factors for cancer-related sleep disturbances are extensive. They include tumor pathophysiology, treatment, adjuvant medications, environment, psychosocial alterations, and comorbid medical conditions.[2] These factors are often categorized as predisposing, precipitating, and perpetuating factors, as described in Spielman and colleagues'[27] 3 P model. **Box 1** outlines the most common risk factors in the context of cancer.

Predisposing Factors

Predisposing factors are enduring psychological or biological traits that increase susceptibility to developing sleep problems. They include older age, female sex, hyperarousability, personal or familial history of sleep problems or mood disturbance, and possible genetic factors. Cancer incidence increases with age[28] and age-related decrements in sleep quality are a predisposing risk factor in many patients with cancer.[7]

Precipitating Medical Factors

Precipitating factors include diseases, treatments, psychological and environmental influences, and life events that trigger sleep disturbances. Progressive tumor growth can increase pressure/pain, impair breathing, and obstruct major organs, leading to disrupted sleep.[19] Cancer treatments that alter inflammatory cytokines or corticosteroid levels (eg, interferon, interleukin-2)[29] may disrupt circadian rhythms and alter mood.[19] Adjunct medications such as opioids and antiemetic corticosteroids disrupt sleep structure and quality.[21] Physical and emotional pain have been linked to delayed sleep onset, frequent awakenings, and poor sleep quality.[30–32] Nausea, diarrhea, genitourinary distress, and respiratory problems caused by chemotherapy are among the many treatment side effects associated with sleep disturbance.[2]

Sleep during hospitalization is habitually interrupted by noise and hospital routines, and the absence of light-dark cues may alter usual circadian cycles. Anxiety, sedation, excessive napping, and temperature dysregulation also contribute to altered sleep patterns.[33]

Perpetuating Factors

Perpetuating factors are behaviors (eg, excessive napping) and beliefs (eg, catastrophic thinking about poor sleep) that people adopt to cope with poor sleep, but that can perpetuate sleep difficulties.[27] Maladaptive behaviors that perpetuate poor sleep and fatigue include an irregular sleep schedule, poor nutrition, inactivity, smoking, and lack of moderation in consumption of alcohol, caffeine, and other stimulants.[34,35]

Consequences of Sleep Disturbance

In noncancer populations, sleep disturbances have been associated with adverse physiologic outcomes, including alterations in immune function,[36] metabolism, nitrogen balance, and protein catabolism.[37] Sleep deprivation and disruption are known to diminish cognitive abilities[38] and sleep disturbance can increase pain intensity, depression, and anxiety.[39,40] Delirium is a common, severe complication in hospitalized older adults with cancer, with multifactorial cause, including sleep disturbance.[41,42]

ASSESSMENTS AND DIAGNOSTICS

Tailored interventions and nursing actions should be based on effective assessment of sleep in hospitalized patients.[43] Sleep assessments include brief screening,

Table 1
Potential sleep disorders in critically ill patients with cancer

Sleep Disorder	Characteristics	Risk Factors/Causes
Sleep deprivation	A sufficient lack of restorative sleep over a cumulative period resulting in physical or psychiatric symptoms, and affecting usual performance	Pharmacologic treatments Acute medical, neurologic, and psychiatric disorders ICU environment (noise, lighting) Routine patient care and monitoring activities Pain and other symptoms Inadequate sleep hygiene Acute stressors Other sleep disorders (eg, RLS, OSA)
Insomnia	Transient or chronic difficulty falling asleep, staying asleep, or awakening too early, despite adequate opportunity, condition, and time. Associated with impairment of daytime function	Advanced age Female gender Pharmacologic treatments and substance use Acute medical, neurologic, and psychiatric disorders and treatments (eg, surgery) Pain and other symptoms Inadequate sleep hygiene Acute stressors Other sleep disorders (eg, RLS, OSA)
OSA	Repetitive reduction or cessation of airflow, despite the presence of respiratory efforts, caused by partial or complete upper airway occlusion during sleep	Advancing age Male gender Family history of OSA Menopause symptoms: normally occurring or induced by cancer treatments Excess body weight Snoring Specific craniofacial and oropharyngeal features Smoking and alcohol use Pharmacologic treatments: muscle relaxants, sedatives, anesthetics, opioid analgesics Concurrent medical disorders: androgen therapy, congestive heart failure, neuromuscular disorders, stroke

CSA	Repetitive cessation of airflow during sleep caused by reduction or loss of ventilatory effort; may be primary or secondary to other medical disorders	Cardiac, renal, and neurologic disorders (eg, renal failure, brainstem lesions, head injury, neuromuscular disorders, stroke) Chronic long-acting opioid use High-altitude breathing
Parasomnias	Physical or experiential phenomena that occur during the sleep period that manifest as activation of the skeletal muscles or autonomic nervous system (eg, confusional arousals, nightmares, sleep walking)	Risk factors are related to the specific manifestations: Familial pattern in confusional arousals Risk factors for nightmares include medications (eg, amphetamines, barbiturates, dopamine agonists, antidepressants) and withdrawal from alcohol and REM sleep suppressants
RLS and periodic limb movement	Neurologic disorder characterized by an urge to move legs, or unpleasant sensations of the legs that begin or worsen during periods of inactivity, are relieved by movement	Female gender Iron deficiency anemia Uremia Pregnancy Peripheral neuropathy Parkinson disease Diabetes mellitus Rheumatoid arthritis Alcohol or caffeine Smoking Pharmacologic treatments: antihistamines, neuroleptics, and dopamine antagonists
Circadian rhythm sleep disorders	Caused by recurrent or persistent misalignment between the desired sleep schedule and the circadian sleep-wake rhythm; can be associated with insomnia and excessive daytime sleepiness	Advanced sleep phase disorder that increases with age Irregular sleep-wake rhythm associated with neurologic disorders (eg, dementia)

Abbreviations: CSA, central sleep apnea; OSA, obstructive sleep apnea; REM, rapid eye movement; RLS, restless legs syndrome.
Data from Refs.[33,81,82]

Box 1
Cancer-related risk factors for sleep disturbance

General predispositions

- Female sex
- Advanced age
- Personal/family history of sleep disturbance/disorder or mood disorder
- Hyperarousal trait

Cancer-related precipitating factors

- Treatments: chemotherapy, radiation, surgery, biologic agents, hormonal agents, molecularly targeted agents
- Primary and adjunct treatments side effects: opioids, anxiolytics, antiemetics, antidepressants, corticosteroids
- Symptoms: pain, dyspnea, hot flashes, nausea, diarrhea
- Psychological distress: depression, anxiety
- Environmental disruptions: noise, light, temperature, absence of sleep-wake cues

Perpetuating factors

- Maladaptive behaviors: excessive time in bed, napping, irregular sleep schedule
- Maladaptive beliefs: unrealistic sleep expectations, excessive worry about sleep

Data from Refs.[7,19,21,28,30–33]

subjective, objective, and diagnostic methods. Subjective evaluation refers to patient sleep descriptions; objective data refers to observation and collection of quantitative information.[43]

Subjective Assessments

Although there are a multitude of subjective sleep measures, lengthy or detailed tools are rarely feasible in acute care settings.[33] **Table 2** summarizes selected

Table 2
Interview and self-report assessments for acute cancer care

Sleep Assessments			
Assessment	**Items**	**Description/Notes**	**Sleep Dimensions**
Clinical Sleep Assessment for Adults[44]	7	Brief questions for a clinic appointment	Sleep history, habits, bedtime routine, nocturnal behaviors
Insomnia Sleep Index[45]	7	Subjective insomnia symptoms and consequences in the past 2 wk	Severity and impact of insomnia
Richards-Campbell Sleep Questionnaire[47]	5	Can be completed in 2 min, has been validated in critical care patients	Sleep onset, total sleep time, awakenings, sleep maintenance, sleep adequacy
Verran Snyder-Halpern Sleep Scale[48]	15	Has been used in critical care research	Sleep latency, fragmentation, length, and depth

Data from Refs.[43–45,47,48]

user-friendly clinical tools such as the 7-item Clinical Sleep Assessment for Adults.[44] The 7-item Insomnia Severity Index[45] is a brief and reliable tool with established validity in cancer populations.[46] In a recent review, Hoey and colleagues[43] evaluated sleep assessments for hospital use. They concluded that the Richards-Campbell Sleep Questionnaire[47] is a brief, reliable measure of sleep quality with great potential for use in hospitalized patients because of its ease of use. The Verran Snyder-Halpern Sleep Scale[48] is a more detailed measure of sleep disturbance and total sleep time that has been tested in patients in ICUs.[43]

Objective Assessments

Clinicians can identify the physiologic basis of pain, other sleep-stealing precipitating factors, and side effects of cancer treatment during physical examinations. In addition, a thorough medical history and medication reconciliation may uncover conditions and medications linked with sleep disorders, or combinations of medications that negatively affect sleep.[49]

Potential diagnostic assessments for the acute care environment include polysomnography (PSG), actigraphy, and Bispectral Index (BIS). PSG is the most accurate measure of sleep and uses sleep onset, duration, awakenings, and architecture to map sleep. Although PSG provides comprehensive sleep data, it is expensive and time consuming to administer and interpret.[50] Portable actigraphy devices calculate sleep-wake periods through body movement, and have been used in acutely ill patients, including those with cancer.[5] Using electroencephalographic data from forehead sensors, BIS is a useful measure of sleep depth in critical care environments.[43,51] **Table 3** describes selected objective sleep assessments. Although these diagnostic tools provide excellent sleep information, data usefulness must be balanced with cost.

Table 3
Measures of objective sleep disturbance

Measure	Description
PSG	A diagnostic test usually conducted in a sleep laboratory involving simultaneous recording of multiple physiologic variables during sleep. Sensors measure brain activity (EEG); airflow; respiratory effort; oxygen saturation; electrocardiogram; and eye, jaw, and leg muscle movement. Information is gathered and outputted as waveform tracings, which assist in the diagnosis of sleep disorders. The use of PSG in ICUs is possible but limited by access and cost
BIS[a]	BIS is a measure of the level of consciousness by algorithmic analysis of a patient's EEG on a scale from 0–100 that represents cortical electrical activity (0 indicates cortical silence and 100 is equivalent to fully awake and alert). BIS scores correlate with different stages of sleep
Wrist actigraphy[a]	A device that is usually worn on the wrist to record periods of activity and inactivity over days to weeks. Accelerometer sensors detect gross movement and absence of movement indicates rest or sleep. Actigraphs provide information about sleep latency, periods of nocturnal awakenings, and total minutes of sleep and wake. Limitations in ICU patients include decreased patient movement caused by sedation, restraints, and weakness

Abbreviation: EEG, electroencephalogram.
[a] Denotes current or potential use in the ICU setting.
Data from Refs.[33,43,82,83]

SLEEP TREATMENTS

Although managing sleep in the context of both cancer and intensive care is challenging, there have been numerous empirical studies of pharmacologic and nonpharmacologic interventions to improve sleep in patients with cancer.[19,52–61] Effective strategies are available, which include addressing treatment-related symptoms; consultation with sleep experts; and pharmacologic, nonpharmacologic, and environmental interventions.

Symptom Management

Attentive monitoring and treatment of concurrent symptoms such as pain, nausea, and depression may ameliorate sleep onset and maintenance problems. Management of other sleep disorders, such as sleep apnea, restless legs syndrome, and periodic limb movement disorders, may require referral and treatment by a sleep medicine specialist. Elimination or lower doses of medications with stimulant or sedation as side effects (eg, corticosteroids, opiates, antidepressants, antiemetics, antihistamines) may provide immediate relief from sleep problems. Sleep-disrupting medications should be discontinued when possible, or gradually reduced to achieve desired therapeutic results. The American College of Critical Care Medicine guidelines recommend systematic tapering of sedatives to reduce the risk of sleep-related withdrawal symptoms.[62]

Pharmacologic Interventions

First-line treatment of insomnia is cognitive behavior therapy; however, pharmacologic treatment is indicated for short-term, targeted management of insomnia.[63] Individualized pharmacologic treatment of sleep disturbance in patients with cancer should begin with a comprehensive sleep assessment. Commonly prescribed sleep medications, described in **Table 4**, are based on evidence from research in patients with primary insomnia. Medication use for sleep disturbance in cancer populations is widespread[64] despite the lack of evidence of effectiveness in many phases of cancer care.[65]

US Food and Drug Administration–approved sleep medications include benzodiazepines, nonbenzodiazepine receptor agonists (non-BzRAs), melatonin agonists, and antidepressants.[66] Non-BzRAs have become the most frequently used hypnotic agents to treat onset and maintenance insomnia because of proven efficacy and reduced side effects. Factors in determining appropriate medications include dose and frequency, absorption, half-life, ability to cross the blood-brain barrier, and short-acting versus long-acting formulation.

Risks of pharmacologic therapy include excessive sedation, hypoventilation, and impaired decision making.[66] These risks are amplified in patients with cancer-related renal, hepatic, and pulmonary conditions and older adults. Additional adverse effects in these vulnerable populations include delirium, increased fall risk, and daytime fatigue.[67]

Nonpharmacologic Interventions

Effective nonpharmacologic approaches to improve sleep disturbances may be broadly grouped into 3 areas: cognitive behavioral interventions, complementary therapies, and environmental strategies. Cognitive behavioral interventions, physical activity/early mobility, and mindfulness-based stress reduction (MBSR) have the most substantial evidence of efficacy in patients with cancer,[65] but there is limited application in the acute/intensive care phase of cancer treatment. The efficacy of complementary therapies (eg, relaxation, imagery, meditation, acupuncture, yoga, massage, and psychoeducation) has been tested in small studies of adult patients with cancer; however, these interventions lack sufficient evidence for recommendation in the cancer population.[65]

Cognitive Behavior Therapy for Insomnia

Cognitive behavior therapy for insomnia (CBTI) is a multicomponent approach designed to eliminate perpetuating factors of insomnia by adjusting sleep schedules and addressing maladaptive habits and beliefs about sleep. Several reviews support the efficacy of CBTI for cancer-related insomnia,[19,52,54] but only selected components (eg, sleep scheduling, normalizing circadian rhythms, sleep hygiene, relaxation) may be applicable to the critical care phase of cancer treatment.[68]

Physical Activity

Benefits of physical activity and early mobilization in the ICU include improvement in sleep, fatigue, quality of life, and functional capacity; stress reduction; enhanced recovery; and shorter hospital stay.[23,69,70] Systematic reviews and meta-analyses[53,54] support the general benefit of exercise to improve sleep in adults with cancer. However, additional research is needed to verify the effect of standardized exercise (eg, type, dose, intensity, timing) and early mobilization on sleep disturbance in various patient groups and in acute phases of cancer care.

Mindfulness-Based Stress Reduction

MBSR comprises 3 aspects: (1) paying attention in a particular way and on purpose, (2) being in the present moment, and (3) being nonjudgmental.[71] MSRB has shown beneficial sleep outcomes in patients with cancer in randomized controlled trials[72–75] and a systematic review[57]; however, these studies were not conducted during acute phases of cancer treatment. MBSR has the potential to improve sleep in cancer populations; however, well-designed studies are needed before mindfulness interventions can be recommended for the critical care setting.

Environmental Controls

Most interventions related to hospital environments in patients without cancer focus on 1 or more of the following: noise reduction,[76] diurnal lighting practices,[76,77] uninterrupted sleep periods,[78] and relaxing music.[79] Nursing interventions that reduce ambient stressors in the acute/intensive care setting and increase patient comfort enhanced patients' sleep,[78] but little is known about sleep outcomes in patients with cancer.

Co-Occurring Cancer-Related Fatigue

CRF, a multidimensional experience of persistent exhaustion unrelated to activity and unrelieved by sleep, is a prevalent, distressing consequence of cancer that coexists with sleep disturbance.[21,23] Poor sleep in the course of cancer treatment predicts higher levels of fatigue, even after adjusting for mood disturbance and physical activity levels.[34] Understanding and concurrently treating sleep disturbance and fatigue can lead to improvement in both problems. Like sleep, initial screening for fatigue can lead to early intervention and improved quality of life.[69] Interventions to manage fatigue are multimodal, and may begin with treatment of anemia, depression, or poor nutrition, or pharmacologic (eg, modafinil) and nonpharmacologic approaches (eg, progressive mobility programs to counteract deconditioning).[23,80]

Table 4
US Food and Drug Administration (FDA)–approved medications commonly used for sleep disturbance

Pharmacologic Class	Usual Adult Dose (mg)	Onset (min)	Average Half-Life (h)	General Comments
Benzodiazepines				Prototype class of hypnotics; replaced by newer BzRAs because of more desirable shorter half-life Cautious use in older adults and those with renal or hepatic insufficiency, and untreated sleep apnea Side effects include tolerance, dependency, morning-after sedation, cognitive impairment, rebound insomnia
Triazolam (Halcion)	0.125–0.25	15–30	2–4	
Temazepam (Restoril)	7.5–30	45–60	8–17	
Flurazepam (Dalmane)	15–30	60–120	48–100	
Nonbenzodiazepine Benzodiazepine Agonists				BzRAs have lower risk of rebound insomnia, tolerance, sleep architecture change, and muscle relaxation compared with older benzodiazepines Zolpidem is available in several approved forms: oral, oral extended-release, sublingual, mist (with similar drug absorption and pharmacokinetic profiles) Extended dosing zolpidem CR has initial release and slow release throughout the night Reduced dosage of BzRAs is recommended for older adults
Zaleplon (Sonata)	5–20	20	1–1.5	
Eszopiclone (Lunesta)	1–3	30	1.5–2.5	
Zolpidem (Ambien)	5–10	30	2.5–2.8	
Zolpidem CR (Ambien CR)	6.25–12.5	30	1.6–5.5	
Zolpidem tartrate sublingual (Edluar)	5–10	—	—	
Zolpidem tartrate mist (Zolpimist)	5–10	—	—	
Melatonin Receptor Agonist				Ramelteon has modest efficacy and a good safety profile, minimal abuse and dependence potential. It is associated with multiple drug and food interactions. Side effects include headache, fatigue, dizziness, nausea, respiratory infection. Cautious use in elderly and patients with hepatic impairment
Ramelteon (Rozerem)	8	30	1–5	

Antidepressants				Despite widespread off-label use, most antidepressants are not FDA approved for insomnia except low-dose doxepin (Silenor), which was approved for onset and maintenance insomnia in 2010. Lower doses of amitriptyline (10–25 mg) may be used for sleep when the antidepressant effect is not needed.
TCAs				Antidepressants for insomnia may be clinically justified if sleep disturbance is concomitant with depression
Amitriptyline (Elavil)	10–300	30–60	14–18	TCAs suppress REM sleep; have many drug interactions; and impair cognition, psychomotor performance. Therefore, cautious use in older adults
Doxepin (Sinequan)	1–25	30–60	20–25	Trazodone may increase slow wave sleep and sleep continuity and should not be taken with MAO inhibitors; trazodone affects daytime performance and is associated with cardiac arrhythmias, orthostatic hypertension, priapism
Doxepin (Silenor)	3–6	30	—	
Serotonin Modulating				
Trazodone (Desyrel)	25–100	30–60	4–7	
Melatonin	0.3–10	—	—	Melatonin, an endogenous hormone released by pineal gland (<0.3 mg/d) in response to dim light onset. Exogenous melatonin is available as OTC nutritional supplement, but is not FDA approved and a recommended dose has not been established. Higher doses may cause anxiety and irritability. An initial low dose, 1–3 mg 1 h before bedtime, is usually effective for insomnia. There are limited clinical trial data to support efficacy of exogenous melatonin for insomnia; however, it is often used for insomnia and circadian rhythm disorders, including jet lag. Significant variability in melatonin content in OTC preparations has been reported

Note: Not intended as a prescribing guide.

Abbreviations: BzRAs, benzodiazepine receptor agonists; CR, controlled release; MAO, monoamine oxidase; OTC, over the counter; REM, rapid eye movement; TCAs, tricyclic antidepressants.

Data from Refs.[63,82,84]; and *Adapted from* Matthews EE. Sleep disturbances and fatigue in critically ill patients. AACN Adv Crit Care 2011;22:213–4; with permission.

SUMMARY

This article confirms the high prevalence and serious consequences of sleep disturbances and fatigue in persons during acute cancer care. With increased knowledge of the nature of sleep problems, risk factors, assessment options, and management strategies, nurses are well positioned to promote sleep health.[43]

Practice Implications

Open communication with health care providers has great potential to improve sleep in hospitalized patients with cancer. Patient and family involvement in individualized care planning may maximize the effectiveness of the sleep interventions. Routine use of available assessment tools can facilitate provider detection of underlying sleep disorders and altered sleep quality. Implementing standard screening and management of sleep problems per institutional policy may prevent sleep disturbance or lessen the impact. For instance, early mobility can improve sleep as well as other clinical outcomes. Pharmacologic interventions, prescribed with caution, can supplement cognitive behavioral and environmental interventions.

Future Research

Well-designed, large trials testing the effectiveness of nonpharmacologic interventions for ICU-related sleep disturbance are warranted, particularly in patients with cancer and other populations with unique risk factors. Additional research is needed to evaluate the feasibility and reliability of various sleep assessments. Deepening the pool of knowledge in these areas will enhance providers' ability to make evidence-based decisions in the treatment of sleep disturbances.

REFERENCES

1. Savard J, Ivers H, Villa J, et al. Natural course of insomnia comorbid with cancer: an 18-month longitudinal study. J Clin Oncol 2011;29:3580–6.
2. Dickerson SS, Connors LM, Fayad A, et al. Sleep-wake disturbances in cancer patients: narrative review of literature focusing on improving quality of life outcomes. Nat Sci Sleep 2014;6:85–100.
3. Boonstra L, Harden K, Jarvis S, et al. Sleep disturbance in hospitalized recipients of stem cell transplantation. Clin J Oncol Nurs 2011;15:271–6.
4. Monas L, Csorba S, Kovalyo M, et al. The relationship of sleep disturbance and symptom severity, symptom interference, and hospitalization among Israeli inpatients with cancer. Oncol Nurs Forum 2012;39:E361–72.
5. Hacker ED, Kapella MC, Park C, et al. Sleep patterns during hospitalization following hematopoietic stem cell transplantation. Oncol Nurs Forum 2015;42:371–9.
6. Palesh OG, Roscoe JA, Mustian KM, et al. Prevalence, demographics, and psychological associations of sleep disruption in patients with cancer: University of Rochester Cancer Center-Community Clinical Oncology Program. J Clin Oncol 2010;28:292–8.
7. Sterniczuk R, Rusak B, Rockwood K. Sleep disturbance in older ICU patients. Clin Interv Aging 2014;9:969.
8. Bihari S, Doug McEvoy R, Matheson E, et al. Factors affecting sleep quality of patients in intensive care unit. J Clin Sleep Med 2012;8:301.
9. Chlan LL, Savik K. Contributors to fatigue in patients receiving mechanical ventilatory support: a descriptive correlational study. Intensive Crit Care Nurs 2015;31:303–8.

10. Delaney LJ, Van Haren F, Lopez V. Sleeping on a problem: the impact of sleep disturbance on intensive care patients - a clinical review. Ann Intensive Care 2015;5:3.
11. Friese RS. Sleep and recovery from critical illness and injury: a review of theory, current practice, and future directions. Crit Care Med 2008;36:697–705.
12. Friese RS, Bruns B, Sinton CM. Sleep deprivation after septic insult increases mortality independent of age. J Trauma 2009;66:50–4.
13. Kamdar BB, Needham DM, Collop NA. Sleep deprivation in critical illness: its role in physical and psychological recovery. J Intensive Care Med 2012;27:97–111.
14. Puxty K, McLoone P, Quasim T, et al. Survival in solid cancer patients following intensive care unit admission. Intensive Care Med 2014;40:1409–28.
15. Benz R, Schanz U, Maggiorini M, et al. Risk factors for ICU admission and ICU survival after allogeneic hematopoietic SCT. Bone Marrow Transplant 2014; 49:62–5.
16. Bird GT, Farquhar-Smith P, Wigmore T, et al. Outcomes and prognostic factors in patients with haematological malignancy admitted to a specialist cancer intensive care unit: a 5 yr study. Br J Anaesth 2012;108:452–9.
17. Chima RS, Abulebda K, Jodele S. Advances in critical care of the pediatric hematopoietic stem cell transplant patient. Pediatr Clin North Am 2013;60: 689–707.
18. Siefert ML, Hong F, Valcarce B, et al. Patient and clinician communication of self-reported insomnia during ambulatory cancer care clinic visits. Cancer Nurs 2014; 37:E51–9.
19. Howell D, Oliver TK, Keller-Olaman S, et al. Sleep disturbance in adults with cancer: a systematic review of evidence for best practices in assessment and management for clinical practice. Ann Oncol 2014;25:791–800.
20. Palesh O, Peppone L, Innominato PF, et al. Prevalence, putative mechanisms, and current management of sleep problems during chemotherapy for cancer. Nat Sci Sleep 2012;4:151–62.
21. Ancoli-Israel S, Savard J. Sleep and fatigue in cancer patients. In: Kryger MH, Roth T, Dement WC, editors. Principles and practice of sleep medicine. 5th edition. Philadelphia: Elsevier Saunders; 2011. p. 1416–21.
22. LeBlanc M, Mérette C, Savard J, et al. Incidence and risk factors of insomnia in a population-based sample. Sleep 2009;32:1027–37.
23. Campos MP, Hassan BJ, Riechelmann R, et al. Cancer-related fatigue: a review. Rev Assoc Med Bras 2011;57:211–9.
24. McKinley S, Fien M, Elliott R, et al. Sleep and psychological health during early recovery from critical illness: an observational study. J Psychosom Res 2013; 75:539–45.
25. Bevans MF, Mitchell SA, Marden S. The symptom experience in the first 100 days following allogeneic hematopoietic stem cell transplantation (HSCT). Support Care Cancer 2008;16:1243–54.
26. Rischer J, Scherwath A, Zander AR, et al. Sleep disturbances and emotional distress in the acute course of hematopoietic stem cell transplantation. Bone Marrow Transplant 2009;44:121–8.
27. Spielman AJ, Caruso LS, Glovinsky PB. A behavioral perspective on insomnia treatment. Psychiatr Clin North Am 1987;10:541–53.
28. Milholland B, Auton A, Suh Y, et al. Age-related somatic mutations in the cancer genome. Oncotarget 2015;6:24627–35.

29. Eisenberger NI, Inagaki TK, Mashal NM, et al. Inflammation and social experience: an inflammatory challenge induces feelings of social disconnection in addition to depressed mood. Brain Behav Immun 2010;24:558–63.
30. Berger AM, Visovsky C, Hertzog M, et al. Usual and worst symptom severity and interference with function in breast cancer survivors. J Support Oncol 2012;10: 112–8.
31. Nishiura M, Tamura A, Nagai H, et al. Assessment of sleep disturbance in lung cancer patients: relationship between sleep disturbance and pain, fatigue, quality of life, and psychological distress. Palliat Support Care 2014;13(3):575–81.
32. Sharma N, Hansen CH, O'Connor M, et al. Sleep problems in cancer patients: prevalence and association with distress and pain. Psychooncology 2012;21: 1003–9.
33. Matthews EE. Sleep disturbances and fatigue in critically ill patients. AACN Adv Crit Care 2011;22:204–24.
34. Goedendorp MM, Gielissen MF, Verhagen CA, et al. Development of fatigue in cancer survivors: a prospective follow-up study from diagnosis into the year after treatment. J Pain Symptom Manage 2013;45:213–22.
35. Aitken LM, Burmeister E, McKinley S, et al. Physical recovery in intensive care unit survivors: a cohort analysis. Am J Crit Care 2015;24:33–9 [quiz: 40].
36. Irwin MR, Wang M, Ribeiro D, et al. Sleep loss activates cellular inflammatory signaling. Biol Psychiatry 2008;64:538–40.
37. Steiger A. Endocrine and metabolic changes during sleep. Handb Clin Neurol 2011;98:241–57.
38. Eugene AR, Masiak J. The neuroprotective aspects of sleep. MEDtube Sci 2015; 3:35–40.
39. Brennan MJ, Lieberman JA. Sleep disturbances in patients with chronic pain: effectively managing opioid analgesia to improve outcomes. Curr Med Res Opin 2009;25:1045–55.
40. Cheng KK, Yeung RM. Impact of mood disturbance, sleep disturbance, fatigue and pain among patients receiving cancer therapy. Eur J Cancer Care (Engl) 2013;22:70–8.
41. Bush SH, Leonard MM, Agar M, et al. End-of-life delirium: issues regarding recognition, optimal management, and the role of sedation in the dying phase. J Pain Symptom Manage 2014;48:215–30.
42. Guo Y, Sun L, Li L, et al. Impact of multicomponent, nonpharmacologic interventions on perioperative cortisol and melatonin levels and postoperative delirium in elderly oral cancer patients. Arch Gerontol Geriatr 2016;62:112–7.
43. Hoey LM, Fulbrook P, Douglas JA. Sleep assessment of hospitalised patients: a literature review. Int J Nurs Stud 2014;51:1281–8.
44. Lee KA, Ward TM. Critical components of a sleep assessment for clinical practice settings. Issues Ment Health Nurs 2005;26:739–50.
45. Morin CM. Insomnia: psychological assessment and management. New York: Guilford Press; 1993.
46. Savard MH, Savard J, Simard S, et al. Empirical validation of the insomnia severity index in cancer patients. Psychooncology 2005;14:429–41.
47. Richards KC, O'Sullivan PS, Phillips RL. Measurement of sleep in critically ill patients. J Nurs Meas 2000;8:131–44.
48. Snyder-Halpern R, Verran JA. Instrumentation to describe subjective sleep characteristics in healthy subjects. Res Nurs Health 1987;10:155–63.
49. Stuck BA, Maurer JT. Airway evaluation in obstructive sleep apnea. Sleep Med Rev 2008;12:411–36.

50. Ward TM. Conducting a sleep assessment. In: Redeker NS, McEnany GP, editors. Sleep disorders and sleep promotion in nursing practice. New York: Springer; 2011. p. 53–70.
51. Pisani MA, Friese RS, Gehlbach BK, et al. Sleep in the intensive care unit. Am J Respir Crit Care Med 2015;191:731.
52. Garland SN, Johnson JA, Savard J, et al. Sleeping well with cancer: a systematic review of cognitive behavioral therapy for insomnia in cancer patients. Neuropsychiatr Dis Treat 2014;10:1113–24.
53. Mishra SI, Scherer RW, Geigle PM, et al. Exercise interventions on health-related quality of life for cancer survivors. Cochrane Database Syst Rev 2012;(8):CD007566.
54. Langford DJ, Lee K, Miaskowski C. Sleep disturbance interventions in oncology patients and family caregivers: a comprehensive review and meta-analysis. Sleep Med Rev 2012;16:397–414.
55. Kwekkeboom KL, Cherwin CH, Lee JW, et al. Mind-body treatments for the pain-fatigue-sleep disturbance symptom cluster in persons with cancer. J Pain Symptom Manage 2010;39:126–38.
56. Wanchai A, Armer JM, Stewart BR. Nonpharmacologic supportive strategies to promote quality of life in patients experiencing cancer-related fatigue: a systematic review. Clin J Oncol Nurs 2011;15:203–14.
57. Winbush NY, Gross CR, Kreitzer MJ. The effects of mindfulness-based stress reduction on sleep disturbance: a systematic review. Explore (NY) 2007;3: 585–91.
58. Garcia MK, McQuade J, Haddad R, et al. Systematic review of acupuncture in cancer care: a synthesis of the evidence. J Clin Oncol 2013;31:952–60.
59. Sharma M, Haider T, Knowlden AP. Yoga as an alternative and complementary treatment for cancer: a systematic review. J Altern Complement Med 2013;19: 870–5.
60. Buffart LM, van Uffelen JG, Riphagen II, et al. Physical and psychosocial benefits of yoga in cancer patients and survivors, a systematic review and meta-analysis of randomized controlled trials. BMC Cancer 2012;12:559.
61. Zhang J, Yang KH, Tian JH, et al. Effects of yoga on psychologic function and quality of life in women with breast cancer: a meta-analysis of randomized controlled trials. J Altern Complement Med 2012;18:994–1002.
62. Jacobi J, Fraser GL, Coursin DB, et al. Clinical practice guidelines for the sustained use of sedatives and analgesics in the critically ill adult. Crit Care Med 2002;30:119–41.
63. Becker PM, Somiah M. Non-benzodiazepine receptor agonists for insomnia. Sleep Med Clin 2015;10:57–76.
64. Casault L, Savard J, Ivers H, et al. Utilization of hypnotic medication in the context of cancer: predictors and frequency of use. Support Care Cancer 2012;20: 1203–10.
65. Irwin M, Johnson LA. Putting evidence into practice: a pocket guide to cancer symptom management. Pittsburgh (PA): Oncology Nursing Society; 2014.
66. Buscemi N, Vandermeer B, Friesen C, et al. The efficacy and safety of drug treatments for chronic insomnia in adults: a meta-analysis of RCTs. J Gen Intern Med 2007;22:1335–50.
67. Tamrat R, Huynh-Le MP, Goyal M. Non-pharmacologic interventions to improve the sleep of hospitalized patients: a systematic review. J Gen Intern Med 2014; 29:788.
68. Morin CM, Benca R. Chronic insomnia. Lancet 2012;379:1129–41.

69. Escalante CP, Kallen MA, Valdres RU, et al. Outcomes of a cancer-related fatigue clinic in a comprehensive cancer center. J Pain Symptom Manage 2010;39: 691–701.
70. Coleman EA, Goodwin JA, Kennedy R, et al. Effects of exercise on fatigue, sleep, and performance: a randomized trial. Oncol Nurs Forum 2012;39:468–77.
71. Tusaie K, Edds K. Understanding and integrating mindfulness into psychiatric mental health nursing practice. Arch Psychiatr Nurs 2009;23:359–65.
72. Garland SN, Carlson LE, Stephens AJ, et al. Mindfulness-based stress reduction compared with cognitive behavioral therapy for the treatment of insomnia comorbid with cancer: a randomized, partially blinded, noninferiority trial. J Clin Oncol 2014;32:449–57.
73. Nakamura Y, Lipschitz DL, Kuhn R, et al. Investigating efficacy of two brief mind-body intervention programs for managing sleep disturbance in cancer survivors: a pilot randomized controlled trial. J Cancer Surviv 2013;7:165–82.
74. Andersen SR, Würtzen H, Steding-Jessen M, et al. Effect of mindfulness-based stress reduction on sleep quality: results of a randomized trial among Danish breast cancer patients. Acta Oncol 2013;52:336–44.
75. Lengacher CA, Kip KE, Barta M, et al. A pilot study evaluating the effect of mindfulness-based stress reduction on psychological status, physical status, salivary cortisol, and interleukin-6 among advanced-stage cancer patients and their caregivers. J Holist Nurs 2012;30:170–85.
76. Yazdannik AR, Zareie A, Hasanpour M, et al. The effect of earplugs and eye mask on patients' perceived sleep quality in intensive care unit. Iran J Nurs Midwifery Res 2014;19:673.
77. Huang HW, Zheng BL, Jiang L, et al. Effect of oral melatonin and wearing earplugs and eye masks on nocturnal sleep in healthy subjects in a simulated intensive care unit environment: which might be a more promising strategy for ICU sleep deprivation? Crit Care 2015;19:124.
78. Eliassen KM, Hopstock LA. Sleep promotion in the intensive care unit—A survey of nurses' interventions. Intensive Crit Care Nurs 2011;27:138.
79. Hu RF, Jiang XY, Hegadoren KM, et al. Effects of earplugs and eye masks combined with relaxing music on sleep, melatonin and cortisol levels in ICU patients: a randomized controlled trial. Crit Care 2015;19:115.
80. Bower JE. Cancer-related fatigue–mechanisms, risk factors, and treatments. Nat Rev Clin Oncol 2014;11:597–609.
81. Bloom HG, Ahmed I, Alessi CA, et al. Evidence-based recommendations for the assessment and management of sleep disorders in older persons. J Am Geriatr Soc 2009;57:761–89.
82. Kryger MH, Roth T, Dement WC. Principles and practice of sleep medicine. New York: Elsevier; 2011.
83. Bourne RS, Minelli C, Mills GH, et al. Clinical review: sleep measurement in critical care patients: research and clinical implications. Crit Care 2007;11:226.
84. National Cancer Institute. Sleep disorders for health professionals (PDQ). Available at: http://www.cancer.gov/about-cancer/treatment/side-effects/sleep-disorders-hp-pdq. Accessed March 3, 2016.

Printed and bound by CPI Group (UK) Ltd, Croydon, CR0 4YY
03/10/2024
01040390-0009